I0788818

Julia R. Seidler

LIVING WITH THE ENEMY

How Chemical Toxins in your Home Affect your Health

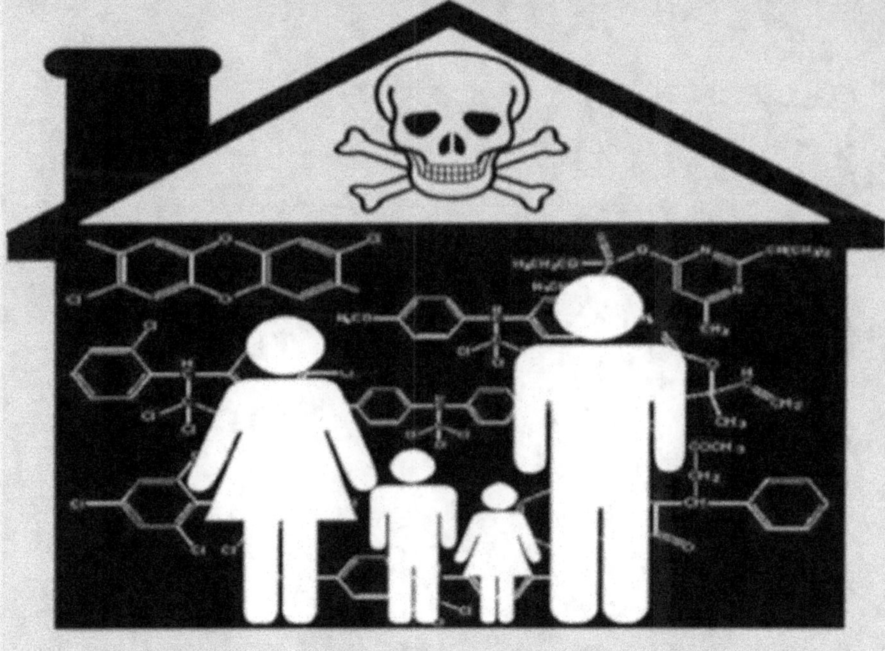

Living With The Enemy

HOW CHEMICAL TOXINS IN YOUR HOME AFFECT YOUR HEALTH

...

Julia R. Seidler

Translated with commentary by Dr. Ramon J. Seidler

ISBN: 1976140471
ISBN 13: 9781976140471

Disclaimer

• • •

The information provided in this book is designed to provide useful information on the topics covered. This book is not intended to be used, nor should it be used, to diagnose or treat any medical condition. For the diagnosis or treatment of any medical problem, consult your doctor. The publisher, editor, translator, and the author are not responsible for any health conditions including allergies that may require medical supervision nor for any damages or negative consequences of any treatment, action, application or preparation, developed after reading the information in this book. References are provided for informational purposes only and do not constitute endorsement of any website or other sources. Readers should be aware that any website that appears in this book may change or become deleted. Some of the websites offer translations.

Dedication

...

I dedicate this book first to God for granting me the knowledge contained in this book and the ability to complete this project. I also dedicate it to my parents for teaching me discipline and the values that guided me through the preparation of this book. Finally, I dedicate this book to my children, Kenneth, Heidy, and Lara, as well as to Edder, and Adita, with the love of both mother and mother-in-law.

Acknowledgements

• • •

I THANK MY DEAR HUSBAND, Ramon Seidler, for his excellent suggestions and his encouragement throughout this project as well as for taking on the English translation and contributing to this book. I also thank Ms. Guitta Karubian (gk@gkwriter.com) for her untiring patience and her professional editorial skills.

Table of Contents

Introduction

· · ·

Exposure to dangerous chemicals is a part of our daily lives. They are present where we work and where we live. They are in the air we breathe, the food we eat, in our water, in the soil, and thus, unfortunately, in our bodies. The amount of chemicals found in some households is alarming and, surprisingly, has little to do with how often the home is cleaned or with its level of maintenance.

The many products present in our homes and in our work areas contain chemicals released into our environment on a daily basis, which can harm our health and the health of our families whether exposed to them on a short or long term basis.

We live in what may be called the *technosphere*. Since the Second World War, the United States has seen the creation of over 85,000 synthetic (man-made) chemicals with both the production and the effects of many of these chemicals too often escaping the attention of regulatory officials, leaving their safety and registration considerations unacknowledged. We are now only beginning to understand how very dangerous some of these chemicals are. The danger is magnified when – as is too often the case – we experience prolonged exposures to numerous chemicals simultaneously.

The chemical world of today has grown exceedingly complex. Chemicals are now interacting with other chemicals as well as with various life forms in unpredictable ways, which in turn result in numerous, unpredictable, and, most often, undesirable, health consequences. Scientists involved with medical research are discovering that continual exposure to this technosphere or "chemical soup" on a daily basis seriously affects the health of both humans and animals around the world. In Europe, medical professionals estimate that chemicals that disturb the body's hormones, known as "endocrine disruptors," are associated with some $200 billion in annual medical costs and lost work time. Recent estimates for the U.S. place the number considerably over $300 billion. [1,2]

Noted scientists at Harvard's School of Public Health have declared that a silent pandemic of neurological illnesses appears to be developing on a global scale. These illnesses are largely associated with exposures to synthetic chemicals including plastics, pesticides, and solvents, as well as some heavy metals that affect both neurological and physical development, especially in children.[3]

The silent nature of the numerous disorders and illnesses caused by exposure to what are called hormone or endocrine disruptors is due to the fact that there is often a significant delay between the exposure to the chemical and its negative effect. Sometimes, it may develop in utero; where exposure occurs in adolescence, the effect may not be expressed until later in life.

These toxic chemicals are often encountered in building materials such as insulation and paints, in plastics and coatings, in air fresheners, perfume fragrances, cleaning and personal hygiene products, tap water, food, household and agricultural pesticides, garden chemicals, electronics, furniture, carpets, and many other items present in our indoor areas. Together they form a very complex cocktail of chemicals which end up accumulating in our bodies. Various international agencies, including the World Health Organization (WHO), recognize that chemical contamination in the home is a serious public health problem for which action is needed. Considering that the western population spends an average of 90% of time indoors, much of which is in the home, the problem becomes obvious.

This book, written for the layperson, describes some of these chemicals and explains how they become toxic, where they may be found within your home and at work, and how you can reduce – or preferably, avoid – your exposure to them.

It behooves us to keep in mind that the toxicity of a substance usually depends upon the dosage. Paracelsus (1493-1541) noted, "The dose makes the difference between a medicine and a poison." However, with the chemicals that are referred to in the 1991 Racine conference, the so-called endocrine disruptors may not adhere to this age old widely accepted concept about toxic chemicals. Also of key importance to toxicity is the degree and length of exposure, the means by which the chemical enters the body, and the state of health of the person among other factors.

For Further Reading

1. https://www.ncbi.nlm.nih.gov/pmc/articles/PMC4399291/
2. http://nyulangone.org/press-releases/yearly-exposure-to-chemicals-dangerous-to-hormone-function-burdens-americans-with-hundreds-of-billions-in-disease-costs
3. https://www.forbes.com/sites/alicegwalton/2014/02/15/11-toxic-chemicals-afffecting-brain-development-in-children/#60e0f07d42a8

CHAPTER 1

Is Your Home Contaminated?

...

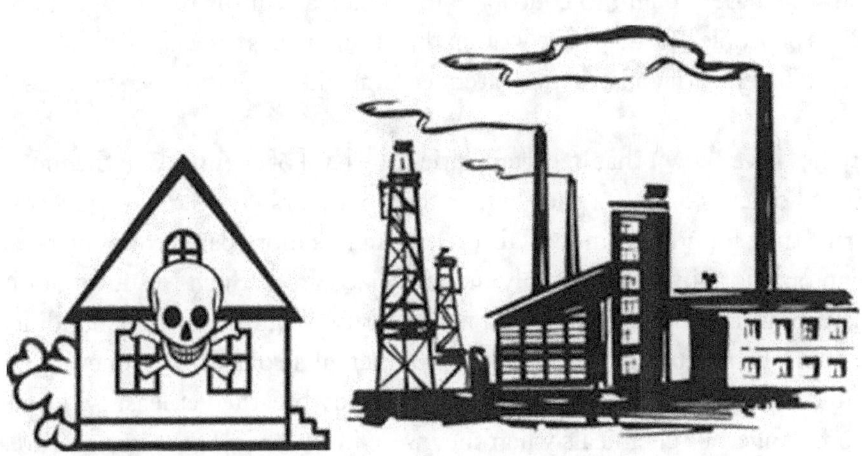

CONTAMINATION FROM CHEMICALS IN THE home has been gradually increasing and has accelerated significantly over the last 60 years with the signaling in of the "Golden Age of Capitalism," a period marked by both economic prosperity and fossil fuel-based industrialization. Today, synthetic materials containing numerous chemicals are used in the construction of new homes and buildings, as well as in the manufacture of many modern necessities of life. Most of these chemicals are toxic. Many (like plastics) are derived from petroleum-based products (like soaps, fragrances, and flooring) or produced through contemporary commercial chemical methodologies.

We spend up to 90% of our time indoors, both at work and in our homes. It is, therefore, extremely important to keep the air and floors in these places as devoid as possible from chemicals that damage our health.

According to an article by Dr. Hector E. Solorzano del Rio (Professor of Pharmacology at the University of Guadalajara and President of the Medical Society of Enzyme Research, AC,[1] "Concerns are growing daily over the toxicity from low level chronic exposures within households and closed workspaces, which produce symptoms that are often caused by unseen pollution, and which are thought to contribute to an increase in the rate of aging processes of people." Others have written that health issues associated with homes should begin with construction, architectural and restoration perspectives.[2]

Studies have shown that in certain cities, the level of chemicals in the indoor air of homes is 5 to 10 times higher than outdoors.[3] Indeed, a recent, long term study found that indoor air often contains more dangerous chemicals than outdoor air even in highly industrialized areas. Such results are quite disturbing since most of us spend the majority of our lives inside buildings. A study conducted by the US Environmental Protection Agency (EPA) found that in a typical day, people in the study breathed at least two times more dangerous chemicals when they were inside their home or work area, compared to the outside area – as for example, in a garden.

Dr. Llewellyn of the Building Research Establishment (BRE) In Great Britain conducted similar studies, reaching the same conclusions as those conducted in North America. He found more than 200 chemicals present in indoor air, 80 of which had significant adverse health consequences. To reduce such chronic and potentially harmful exposures and offset such health problems, it has been recommended that homes in England undergo a complete exchange of air every two hours.

In 1978, the great pioneer of Clinical Ecology, Theron Randolph, studied allergies and human sensitivity to substances in the environment and was the first to describe a human disease that caused an overload in the body's ability to detoxify invisible indoor environmental pollutants. He called the syndrome *multiple chemical sensitivity* (MCS), a "chronic, recurring disease caused by a person's inability to tolerate an environmental chemical or class of foreign chemicals." Ross described this syndrome in further detail in 1997 and presented information that exposure to toxic chemicals can have effects on brain functioning.[4] Although simple and intermittent chemical exposures may not cause acute damage in the short-term, if exposure to these chemicals is repeated daily in the home for prolonged periods of time, the body's defense systems will eventually fail to prevent the onset of long term or chronic illnesses.

What Products in Your Home Contain Harmful Chemicals?

Toxic chemical substances incorporated into everyday household items are released into the environment in various ways. Let's look at some specific examples.

Cleaning Products

Products made for household cleaning, including detergents and disinfectants, contain hazardous chemicals such as ammonia, sulfuric and phosphoric acid, caustic soda, chlorine, formaldehyde, and phenol. Most window and glass cleaners contain ammonia, a highly toxic chemical, which irritates the skin, eyes, nasal passages, and, when inhaled, can be highly corrosive to the respiratory system.

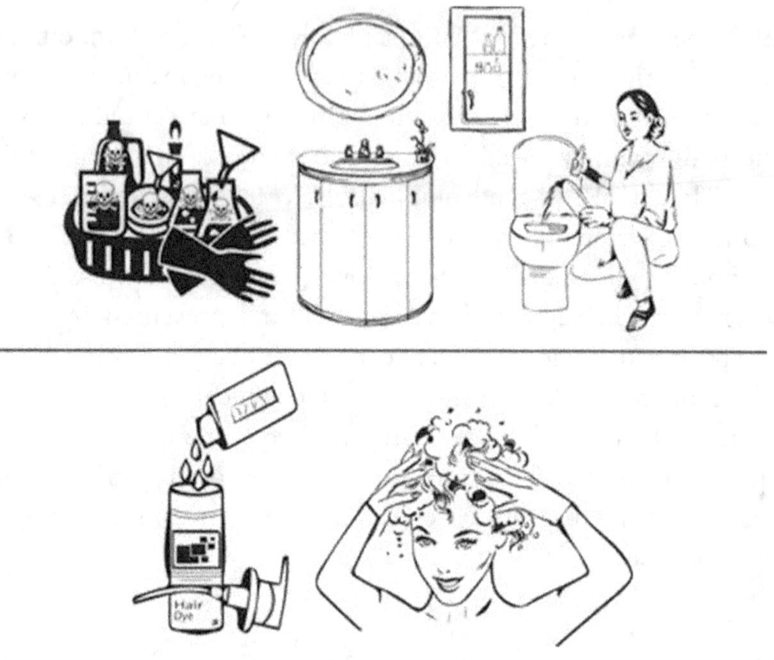

Hair Dyes

Ammonia is also present in the formulas for hair dyes used both in salons and at home. Prolonged exposure to ammonia often causes "olfactory fatigue" or adaptation, making its presence difficult to detect when exposure is prolonged.[5]

Air Fresheners and Fragrances

Most "air fresheners" like car air fresheners, sprays, candles, and oils currently on the market are manufactured from artificial fragrances. These products may also contain a variety of other toxic chemicals in their formulations such as phthalates emitted with each use. Phthalates are associated with cancers and hormonal disorders (i.e., endocrine disruption), and are especially dangerous to the reproductive system causing disorders as discussed below and in this study from the Environmental Working Group.[6]

It has also been observed that when oil-based air fresheners are regularly inhaled, they can form a layer of oil in the nasal passages that contains methoxychlor, an endocrine disrupting pesticide. Like prolonged or repeated exposure to ammonia, methoxychlor may inactivate the nerves of the nose and interfere with the ability to perceive odors over time (known as "olfactory fatigue"). In other words, rather than removing or replacing objectionable odors from the air, some fragrances and air fresheners actually work by adding toxic chemicals into the air, which deaden the ability to perceive the odor.[7]

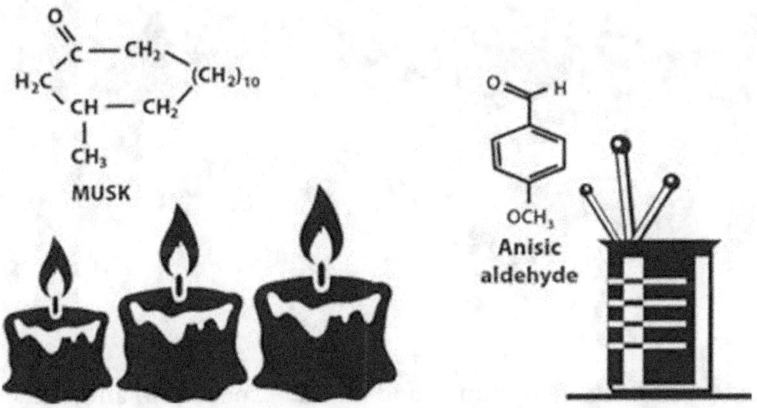

According to a series of studies, artificial fragrances are also a major cause of "cosmetic contact dermatitis," a rash that presently affects more than two million people.[8] Environmental researchers have detected synthetic fragrances in ocean fish and shellfish as well as other aquatic organisms by which one may infer that these chemicals are not readily decomposed but rather, pass through wastewater treatment facilities into environmental waters largely unmodified. Components in some fragrances can even interfere with the transport of proteins through cell membranes, an otherwise natural process needed to remove toxins from the cells.[9]

Adding fragrances to a multitude of products has created a lucrative business in the marketing and advertising laboratories of the cosmetics industry. They hide the ingredients used in their products, which is allowed by law, in every country where their products are sold.

PERSONAL CARE AND HYGIENE PRODUCTS

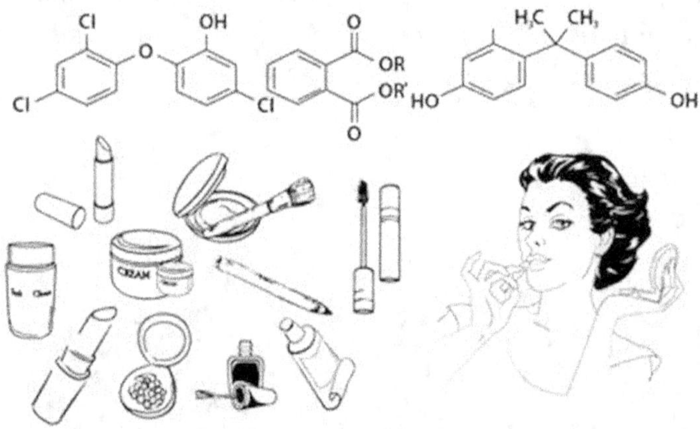

The extent of dangerous human and animal exposure to any of the 3,100 potentially toxic ingredients in personal care items, soaps, and fragrance products is unimaginable. These chemicals are with us continually, and should be a major source of health concerns to us all.[10]

The image above shows examples of cosmetics and personal hygiene products that could be contaminated with toxic endocrine disrupting chemicals. Most of these products are soaps, antibacterial gels, hair shampoos, skin creams, toothpaste and cosmetics that contain a chemical called "triclosan," marketed as "the answer to stop the spread of germs." In reality, triclosan has actually been responsible for widespread resistance of germs to antibiotics and the ensuing production of "supergerms" that have become resistant to various antibiotics.

PESTICIDES

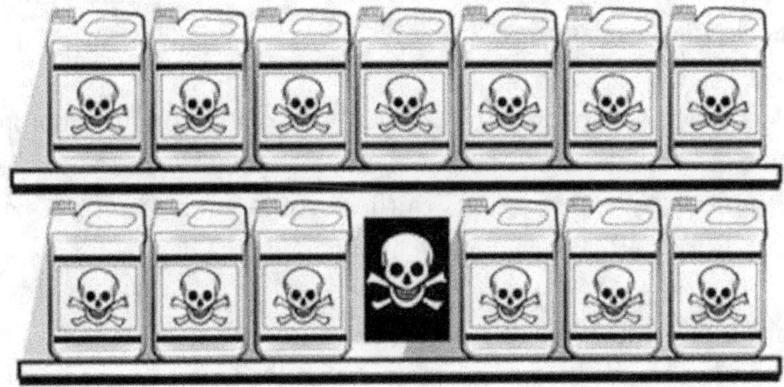

Most pesticides used in the home are not natural; rather, they are manufactured and thus, of synthetic origin. There are currently more than five hundred synthetic pesticides marketed for home and garden use to kill pests, e.g. weeds, insects, fungi, etc. These products are often used carelessly and indiscriminately by the homeowner, resulting in unintended exposures within the home to family members and pets. When used outside, these toxic products are exposed to the natural ecosystems detrimentally affecting wildlife, fish, and beneficial insects, including pollinators. When pesticides are used in commercial agriculture, these toxic chemicals wind up in our foods.

DDT, glyphosate, 2,4-D, atrazine, dieldrin, aldrin, heptachlor, and chlorpyrifos are among the most widely used synthetic pesticides in the world. To the surprise of most Americans, DDT – though not used within the U.S. – is still manufactured in at least 3 countries (North Korea, India, and China) and is used on a "will use as needed" list by at least 31 additional countries.[11]

Chemicals in the Air From Construction and Home Decoration

Chronic exposure to toxic gaseous pollutants known as Volatile Organic Compounds (VOCs) in the indoor environment have been linked to a number of diseases ranging from simple allergies, sinusitis, asthma, headache, fatigue, anxiety, and insomnia to more serious syndromes involving multiple chemical sensitivities.[12]

Career painters occupationally exposed to volatile organic compounds on a continuing basis were found to be significantly more predisposed to adverse neurological reactions to these compounds than non-painters, including serious diseases such as "chronic painter's syndrome."[13]

Some major sources of volatile organic compounds include the following:

A) Building materials such as paints, varnishes, caulks, flooring;

B) Wood finishing elements such as varnishes, polyurethanes, lacquers, and shellac, which may emit significant amounts of VOCs. Even some "natural" oils (eg., linseed and tung oils) may contain petroleum based VOC thinners and/or heavy metals.[14] Personal care products such as air fresheners, cleaning products, and cosmetics;

C) Miscelaneous sources such as second-hand smoke, photocopiers, gasoline, and burning of wood.[15]

Products designed for office use and use in construction contain volatile organic compounds (VOCs) and/or other toxic chemicals. Multiple materials used for home construction (wood flooring, paints, etc.) and items used for home decoration (furniture and decorative elements) liberate toxic substances such as volatile organic compounds (VOCs), constantly releasing them into the environment.

Carpets, curtains, paint, wall paper, and some furniture also release VOCs. Other synthetic materials associated with furniture, foams, leatherettes, wood flooring materials all contain toxic substances such as flame retardants, formaldehyde, and other toxic chemicals found in house dust.[16]

Wooden furniture may also contain undesirable compounds such as toxic preservatives or varnishes that release their toxic VOC substances into the home environment. Wooden patio furniture and fencing are also likely to be specially treated with VOCs and pesticide chemicals to make them resistant to rain and termites. The gypsum boards, glued wood composites and plywood panels that cover roofs and walls and sometimes floors, release various toxic substances like formaldehyde as do insulation materials.

Other construction materials like adhesives, paints, and marking pens should be handled in areas that are adequately ventilated. Continued and inappropriate use of these products make our home a hazardous environment, especially for unsuspecting infants, young children, the elderly, and inside pets like birds, fish, dogs, and cats.

PLASTICS

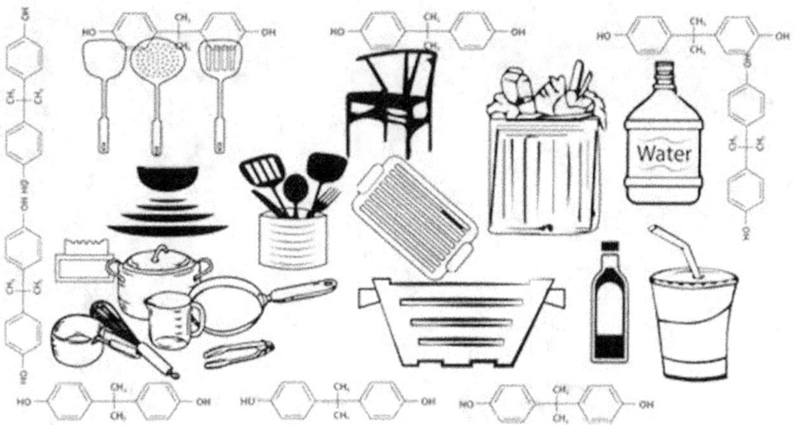

Plastics contain an assortment of potentially toxic chemicals. Polyvinyl chloride (PVC) is a plastic substance that is usually found in shower curtains, food containers, lunch boxes, children's toys, vinyl flooring, plumbing, and many other items. PVC is a toxic substance that has been labeled as "carcinogenic" by the World Health Organization.

Nearly all plastic materials have also been treated with chemical plasticizers made from hazardous materials. Phthalates are a common softening agent for otherwise brittle plastics.

Plastics and Children's Toys

Children's toys are often made from plastics that contain endocrine disrupting chemicals. Phthalates are generally used in the manufacture of most soft plastic toys for children. A recent study by the Public Interest Research Group (PIRG) also found that substances present such as phthalates, lead and chromium were above the legal limits in some toys. These chemicals are linked to allergies, cancers, and male reproductive developmental problems.[17]

The longer children play with plastic toys and particularly when inserting them into their mouth, the greater their exposures to toxic materials and the greater the risk to their health.

Plastic baby bottles and pacifiers

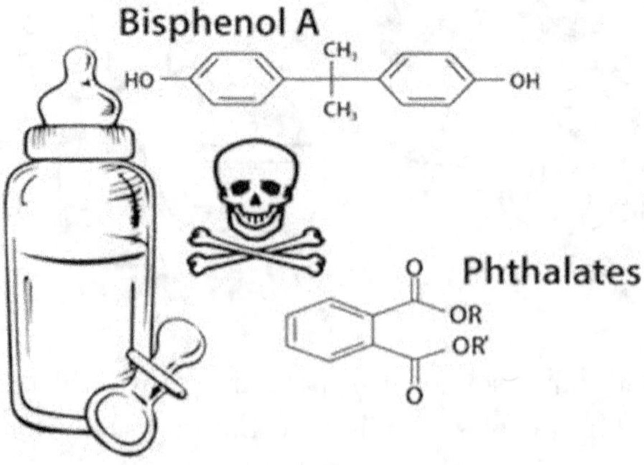

Baby bottles and pacifiers may contain toxic Bisphenol A and/or phthalates. Bisphenol-A (or BPA), is a synthetic chemical and hormone disruptor, which can be found in almost any plastic material, including some nipples in baby bottles, plastic toys for children and babies, plastic containers for food storage and even water supply pipes made of PVC. Carcinogenic PVC is lined with the endocrine disruptor Bisphenol A resulting in double exposure to toxics for anyone daily consuming water emanating from such pipes commonly used within the home.

Plastic food containers

Plastic food storage containers may contain Bisphenol A. It is very easy for Bisphenol A to leak into foods put in plastic containers especially when heated. It is preferable to use stainless steel containers or quality glass to store and cook food. When the use of plastic is mandatory, choose products labeled "free of BPA" for safety and always check the recycling label. Knowing the recycling number provides a way to avoid plastics containing toxic chemicals.

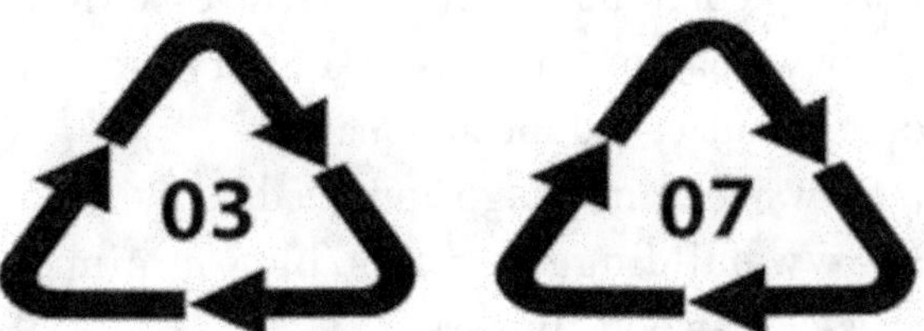

When a recycling label contains the number 03 it means that the plastic contains a phthalate and/or PVC while a 07 within a triangle, indicates the presence of BPA and is also likely to contain other toxic chemicals since 07 is a catch all designation and such plastics should be avoided. Some recycling companies will not accept plastics numbered 3 or 7.

For Further Reading Chapter 1

1. http://www.hector.solorzano.com.mx/032.html
2. https://www.amazon.com/Prescriptions-Healthy-House-3rd-Architects/dp/0865716048
3. http://www.sciencedirect.com/science/article/pii/S0013935187800300
4. https://www.ncbi.nlm.nih.gov/pmc/articles/PMC1469809
5. http://www.atsdr.cdc.gov/mmg/mmg.asp?id=7&tid=2
6. http://mamavation.com/2015/03/toxic-perfume-chemicals.html
7. http://ac.els-cdn.com/S0360132316304334/1-s2.0-S0360132316304334-main.pdf?_tid=662b08e4-6b69-11e7-8dfd-00000aab0f6c&acdnat=1500348788_9bb8f2d9d1fbff69e5048301b3a05b01
8. http://www.webmd.com/allergies/features/fragrance-allergies-a-sensory-assault#1
9. https://www.epa.gov/fish-tech/pilot-study-pharmaceuticals-and-personal-care-products-fish-tissue
10. https://www.nontoxic.com/nontoxic/
11. https://www.ncbi.nlm.nih.gov/pmc/articles/PMC3138025/
12. https://www.epa.gov/indoor-air-quality-iaq/volatile-organic-compounds-impact-indoor-air-quality
13. https://www.ncbi.nlm.nih.gov/pubmed/8472664
14. https://www.buildinggreen.com/blog/minimizing-exposure-chemicals-clear-wood-finishes
15. http://www.health.state.mn.us/divs/eh/indoorair/voc/
16. https://www.theguardian.com/science/2016/sep/14/toxic-chemicals-household-dust-health-cancer-infertility
17. http://www.uspirg.org/reports/usp/trouble-toyland-2015.

CHAPTER 2

Endocrine (Hormone) Disruptors

• • •

AT A 1991 CONFERENCE IN Racine Wisconsin, an international panel made up of 21 scientists declared for the first time ever, they were certain that, "a large number of man-made chemicals have been released into the environment, as well as a few natural ones, which have the potential to disrupt the endocrine system of animals, including humans." These chemicals included pesticides, industrial chemicals, and other synthetic products. They went on to assert,

> *"Many wildlife populations are already affected by these compounds. The impacts include thyroid dysfunction in birds and fish; decreased fertility in birds, fish, shellfish, and mammals; decreased hatching success in birds, fish and turtles; gross birth deformities in birds, fish, and turtles; metabolic abnormalities in birds, fish, and mammals; behavioral abnormalities in birds; demasculinization and feminization of male fish, birds and mammals; defeminization and masculinization of female fish and birds; and compromised immune systems in birds and mammals."*

The panel stated, "Humans may be at risk to the same environmental hazards as wildlife."[1]

How Do Chemicals in Your Home Cause Hormonal Problems?

Prolonged exposure to many of the chemicals described in this book affect the hormonal (endocrine) system of both animals and humans, producing many irreversible illnesses and diseases. The damage to the endocrine system is due to the fact that certain toxic substances have a chemical structure similar to those of natural hormones especially in regard to their chemical ring structure.

These toxic chemicals target natural hormone receptor sites inside cells. When these chemicals interact with the target sites, they can slow down, stop, or stimulate normal bodily functions at inappropriate times resulting in illness or a disease process that is sometimes delayed, sometimes chronic and lifelong. It depends upon the individual hormone and which life process is affected, at what stage of life the interaction occurs, and the extent or longevity of the toxic hormone interaction.

The Hormonal (Endocrine) System

The hormonal or endocrine system consists of a set of critical body organs and tissues that release minute amounts of a natural chemical called a hormone. In the following figure we can observe where these hormones are produced.

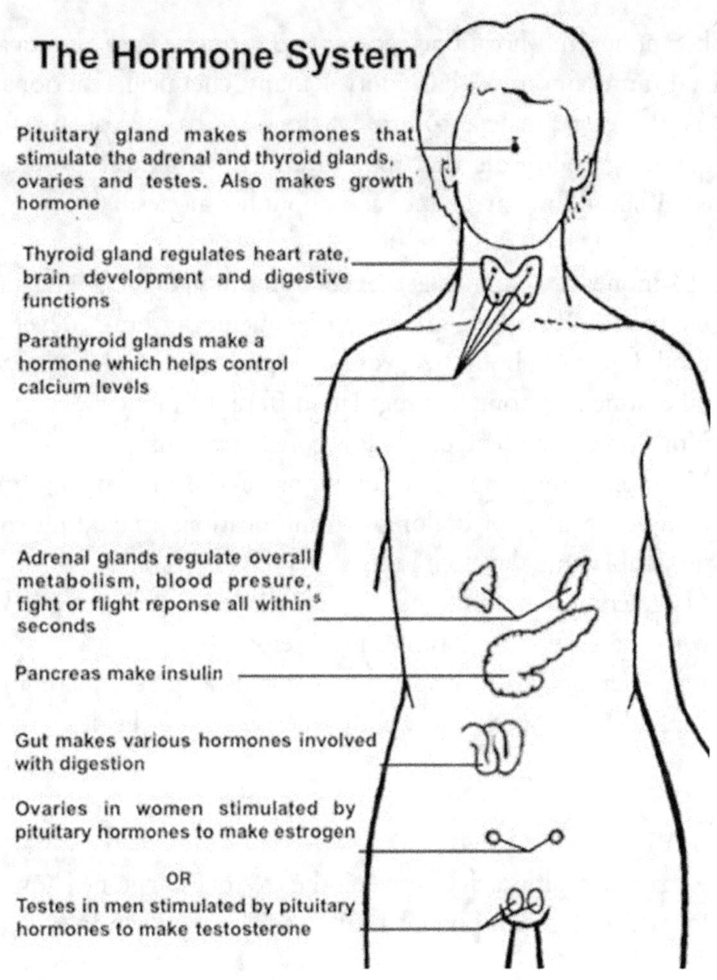

Reproduced with permission from patient.co.uk, Gemma Grange

HORMONES: THEIR FUNCTIONS AND CHARACTERISTICS

The endocrine system is responsible for regulating all major bodily functions of the organism. The hormones, produced by the collection of glands shown above, regulate metabolism, growth and physical development, mental development including a role in determining I.Q., tissue function, sexual function, reproduction, sleep, mood, etc. The system consists of glands, hormones and hormone receptors. Hormones are chemicals produced in minute amounts that control many chemical reactions in the body. It is, therefore, crucial to protect the body from exposure to endocrine disrupting chemicals that may interfere with these processes and reactions. What follows are some facts about hormones:

* Hormones are chemicals that act as messengers triggering numerous bodily functions and activities including brain development, food digestion, body size, sperm production, ovulation, etc;
* The same hormone can regulate different functions;
* Hormones act at extremely low concentrations;
* Hormones regulate vital functions of the organism, through a complex system of lifelong communications, including throughout embryonic development;
* Many components of the endocrine system often act in concert with the nervous and immune system;
* Each person has a different hormonal balance and requirement depending upon age, sex, body weight, general health, etc.

THE THYROID HORMONE

Note the structural similarity between the thyroid hormone shown below and triclosan, Bisphenol A and even fire retardants shown in Chapter 3.

Thyroid hormone T3

Notice the three atoms of iodine (**I**).

Only the thyroid gland is capable of removing iodine from foods and converting it into the "thyroid hormone." The thyroid's iodinated hormones regulate numerous vital body functions, including:

* Breathing
* Heart rate
* Central and peripheral nervous systems
* Body weight
* Muscle strength
* Menstrual cycles
* Body temperature
* Cholesterol levels and more[2]

Testosterone

Testosterone, the primary male sex hormone, plays a crucial role in the development of male reproductive tissues such as the testis and prostate, as well as promoting other sexual characteristics such as increased muscle and bone mass, and the growth of body hair.

Norepinephrine, also known as Adrenaline

Norepinephrine (nickname, adrenaline) is produced in the brain and adrenal gland. It is a truly remarkable multifunctional hormone that reaches highest levels during situations of stress or danger, and is the chemical basis for the so-called "fight-or-flight response." In the brain, norepinephrine increases arousal and alertness, promotes vigilance, and enhances formation and retrieval of memory. In the rest of the body, norepinephrine increases heart rate and blood pressure, triggers the release of glucose from energy stores, increases blood flow to skeletal muscle, reduces blood flow to the gastrointestinal system, and inhibits voiding of the bladder and gastrointestinal movement.[3]

Estradiol is estrogen (page 38), the primary female hormone. Estradiol is essential for the development and maintenance of female reproductive tissues such as the breasts, uterus, and vagina during puberty, adulthood, and pregnancy. It also has an important effect on many other tissues including bone, fat, skin, liver, and the brain. Found at lower levels, estrogen also has special important functions in men as well.[4]

What are Endocrine Disruptors (EDs)?

Endocrine disruptors are chemicals that may interfere with the body's endocrine (hormone) system and produce adverse developmental, reproductive, neurological, and immune effects in both humans and wildlife.[5]

The study and identification of endocrine disruptors is a relatively new field of science.

The term "endocrine disruptor" was first proposed at a conference organized by Dr. Theo Colborn of the World Wildlife Fund in Wisconsin, in 1991. The aim of that conference was to analyze available evidence on the effect of environmental pollutants on the endocrine system of wild animals.

Exposure to chemical EDs can occur in your home and in your workplace, through environmental contamination, including food contaminated with pesticides, exposure to plastic products and plasticizers, and the use of cleaning products. Harmful effects can occur at very low doses, generally well below the legally established exposure limits.

There are numerous kinds of endocrine disruptors with many different chemical structures (see four synthetic EDs below). There are both natural and artificial (synthetic) EDs and they are present everywhere in our surroundings, as documented in a large number of published articles including this book.

SOME UNIQUE CHARACTERISTICS OF ENDOCRINE DISRUPTORS:

- They can act at very low doses (parts per billion or less).
- There are periods of human development such as early pregnancy when the fetus is especially vulnerable to endocrine disruption, causing damage that can lead to significant health effects throughout life.
- The dose-effect relationship of EDs is not linear as it is with most toxic chemicals.
- They can act by combining with each other.
- Some may produce generational effects.
- They may have long periods of latency.
- Exposure to EDs has no space or time limits.
- So far it has not been possible for regulators to agree on safe exposure thresholds to

EDs. As a result, these EDs are generally not regulated within the U.S., they are just being screened for possible activity.[6]

By altering the hormonal balance of organisms, EDs cause an interruption of many natural physiological processes controlled by hormones, provoking a response of greater or lesser intensity than normal, leaving the hormonal system out of balance with its natural control mechanisms. A non-inclusive list of some examples of endocrine disruptors found commonly in the home include: pesticides, alkyl phenols, Bisphenol-A, dioxins, solvents (e.g. perchlorethylene), styrene, phthalates, PBBs, PCBs, tributyltin (TBT), Biphenyl polychlorides, furniture flame retardants, and volatile organic compounds (VOCs).

Currently Bisphenol A and Phthalates are among the most common endocrine disruptors found in the home. These two substances are present in almost all products made into plastics and thus are the main sources of endocrine disruptors today.

However, many other everyday products also contain chemicals that may cause damage to the hormonal system, such as paper receipts, money, plastic films lining the inside of cans, and electronic components in cell phones, tablets, computers, etc. These are common products that many people use daily, making it difficult (but not impossible) to avoid or reduce contact with EDs.

Some Common Endocrine Disruptors

Isoflavones (Plant Produced)
Isoflavones are a class of natural, plant-derived compounds (phytoestrogens) with estrogenic hormone disruptor activity. Isoflavones are examples of natural, plant produced endocrine disruptors (ED) that alter the amount of estrogen in the body. Such compounds are produced in soybeans and other leguminous plants and are present in many species of nuts, seeds, and plant oils. Phytoestrogens such as isoflavones

can exhibit endocrine disrupting activity and have the potential to affect a wide array of the body's intracellular signaling mechanisms important for regulating cellular growth and protection. However, much scientific research addressing the issues as to whether plant derived natural phytoestrogens are beneficial or harmful is still a very widely debated topic.[7,]

The diagram below shows the chemical structures of natural and synthetic hormone (estrogen) and endocrine disruptors. Genistein, a natural isoflavone (plant estrogen) produced by soy and the natural human estrogen, estradiol are shown.[8]

Natural estrogens

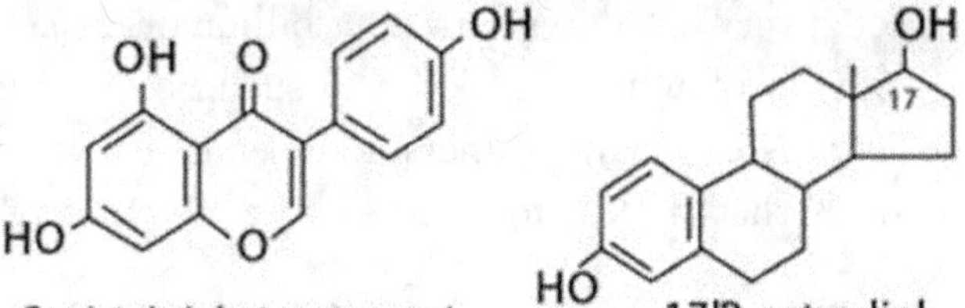

Genistein(phytoestrogen)

17ẞ-estradiol

Four Synthetic Hormone Disruptors

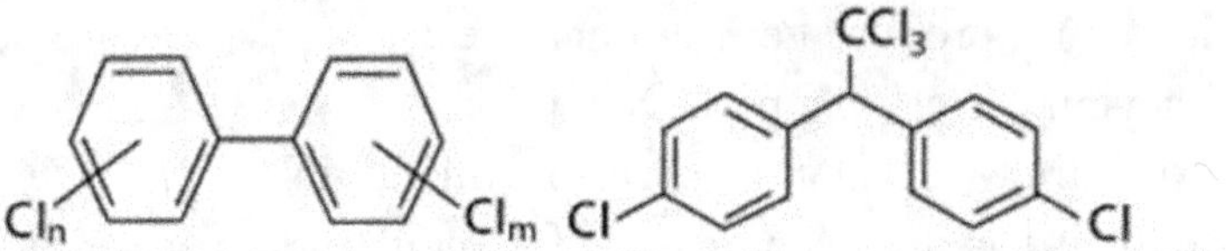

Polychlorinated Biphenyl(PCB)

Dichlorodiphenyltrichloroethane(DDT)

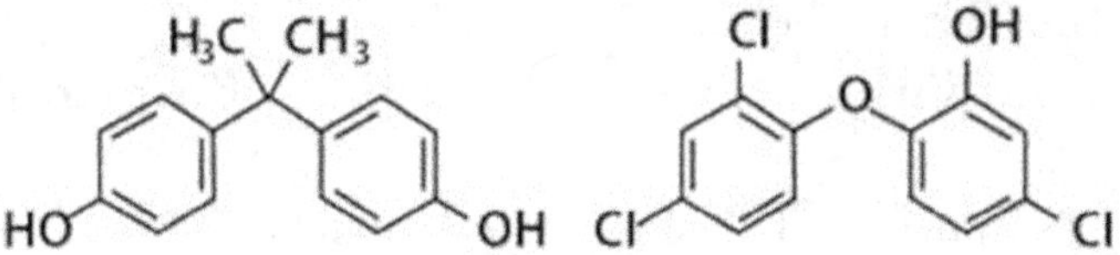

Bisphenol A(BPA)

Triclosan

Synthetic EDs are considered pollutants that cause a variety of problems ranging from infertility and sex changes in fish and laboratory invertebrates taken from water contaminated with these chemicals to serious life-threatening complications in humans.

These ED chemicals do not have a standard of comparison in nature, so they are unique and not included among natural compounds with known hormonal activity.

Generally, synthetic EDs are not produced for therapeutic or diagnostic purposes (except by mistake) and are therefore not classified as residues of medicines or drugs used in human or veterinary medicine.

Among the unique characteristics of endocrine disruptors we can say:

- They can act at very low doses (parts per billion or less).
- There are periods of human development such as early pregnancy when the fetus is especially vulnerable to endocrine disruption, causing damage that can lead to significant health effects throughout life.
- The dose-effect relationship of EDs is not linear as it is with most toxic chemicals.
- They can act by combining with each other.
- Some may produce generational effects.
- They may have long periods of latency.
- Exposure to EDs has no space or time limits.
- So far it has not been possible for regulators to agree on safe exposure thresholds to EDs. As a result these EDs generally, are not regulated within the U.S.[10]
- Endocrine disruptors are present everywhere in our surroundings.

By altering the hormonal balance of organisms, EDs cause an interruption of many natural physiological processes controlled by hormones, provoking a response of greater or lesser intensity than normal, leaving the hormonal system out of balance with natural control mechanisms.

A non-inclusive list of some examples of endocrine disruptors found commonly in the home include: pesticides, alkyl phenols, Bisphenol-A, dioxins, solvents (e.g. perchloroethylene), styrene, phthalates, PBBs, PCBs, tributyltin (TBT), Biphenyl polychlorides, furniture flame retardants, and volatile organic compounds (VOCs).

Bisphenol A and Phthalates

Bisphenol A and Phthalates are among the most common endocrine disrupters in the home that are suspected of causing hormonal imbalances. These two substances are present in almost all products made into plastics and thus are the main sources of endocrine disruptors today. It is important to look for their presence on product labels in daily personal use products and discard or replace them with safer products. However, many other everyday products also contain chemicals that may cause damage to the hormonal system, such as paper receipts, money, plastic films lining the inside of cans, and electronic components in cell phones, tablets, computers, etc. These are common products that many people use daily, making it difficult (but not impossible) to avoid contact with EDs.

What are Some Effects of Endocrine Disruptors?

The balance of the human body metabolic systems depends on the presence of natural chemical mediators (hormones), and the kinds and amounts of endocrine disruptors that interfere with these systems.

Alterations in the male reproductive system

Exposure of the male reproductive system to endocrine disruptors correlates with three effects that are normally considered interrelated:

1. Reduction of reproductive capacity manifested by a decrease in the quality of semen.

2. Impaired fetal development resulting in congenital malformations of the urogenital tract such as cryptorchidism (non-testicular descent) and hypospadias (abnormal position of the opening of the urethra);
3. Emergence of germ cell tumors of the testicles.

ALTERATIONS IN THE FEMALE REPRODUCTIVE SYSTEM

Exposure to endocrine disruptors, especially during fetal development, has been related to:

1. Early onset of puberty.
2. Reduction of fertility due to damage to the eggs and alteration of the menstrual cycle.
3. Polycystic ovarian syndrome: Causes in menstrual changes, infertility, hirsutism (excess hair growth in places normally associated with men), acne, obesity and metabolic syndromes.
4. Fertility problems: Related to spontaneous abortions, ectopic pregnancies, stillbirth, death at birth, preterm delivery, low birth weight, altered sex ratios in the family.
5. Adverse pregnancy problems such as miscarriages, preeclampsia and uterine growth restriction.
6. Endometriosis and uterine fibroids (non-cancerous tumors): Endometriosis is the presence of endometrial tissue outside the uterus, which causes chronic pelvic pain and infertility; uterine fibroids or myomas are benign tumors of myometrium smooth muscle.
7. Breast and ovarian cancer.

EFFECTS ON THE INTELLIGENCE COEFFICIENT (I.Q.)

A recent study suggests that prenatal exposure of pregnant women to certain EDCs could cause the loss of IQ and general intellectual disability associated with autism. The adverse effect on thyroid hormone production by some endocrine disruptors affects brain development in the fetus.[10]

Attention deficit hyperactivity disorder in children has been linked to exposure to insecticidal organophosphates.[11]

Other effects observed in children such as low reading comprehension, low IQ and memory problems have been related to exposure of the fetus to PCBs.[12]

A decrease in the chemical element lithium in the body has an established relationship with depressive states. In laboratory experiments, the ability of the organophosphate pesticides (parathion, chlorpyrifos and methamidophos) to decrease lithium levels in chickens has been demonstrated. In some countries there has been an increase in suicides that have been linked to continued exposure to various pesticides implying that depression may have been related to lowered lithium levels due to organophosphate exposures.

ADDITIONAL ALTERATIONS

1. EDs can alter the concentrations of the natural hormones and enzymes promoting or interfering in the modifications of the liver. This can lead to non-alcoholic fatty liver disease (NAFLD) that in turn may lead to obesity and diabetes.[13]
2. EDCs can alter the number of hormone receptors during tissue development predisposing these tissues to subsequent abnormal processes throughout life.

In any case, it is clear that without a healthy endocrine system, the body and the brain will suffer the consequences of potentially lifelong illnesses with the potential of severe medical and personal costs. Toxic chemicals in the home are truly an international problem of massive proportions.[14]

For Further Reading Chapter 2

1. http://www.ourstolenfuture.org/consensus/wingspread1.htm
2. https://www.endocrineweb.com/conditions/thyroid/how-your-thyroid-works
3. https://en.wikipedia.org/wiki/Norepinephrine
4. https://en.wikipedia.org/wiki/Estradiol
5. https://www.niehs.nih.gov/health/topics/agents/endocrine/index.cfm
6. http://www.chemsafetypro.com/Topics/USA/Endocrine_Disruptor_Regulations_and_Lists_in_USA.html
7. https://www.ncbi.nlm.nih.gov/pmc/articles/PMC3074428/
8. http://lpi.oregonstate.edu/mic/dietary-factors/phytochemicals/soy-isoflavones.
9. https://www.epa.gov/endocrine-disruption/endocrine-disruptor-screening-program-timeline
10. http://www.newswise.com/articles/exposure-to-endocrine-disrupting-chemicals-can-adversely-affect-brain-development
11. https://www.ncbi.nlm.nih.gov/pubmed/27070915
12. http://www.thelancet.com/journals/lancet/article/PIIS0140-6736(01)06654-5/fulltext
13. https://www.sciencedaily.com/releases/2015/03/150306181811.htm
14. https://www.aacc.org/publications/cln/cln-stat/2016/november/17/endocrine-disruptors-cost-us-more-than-340-billion-in-health-and-other-costs

CHAPTER 3

What Principle Chemical Substances in Your Home Cause Health Problems?

• • •

CLASSIFYING CHEMICALS IN YOUR HOME

POLLUTANTS INSIDE THE HOME EXIST in one of three physical states:

1. **Particulate matter**. This includes dust, smoke, pollen and particles generated by combustion appliances, including cooking, as well as biological particles associated with small organisms such as mites, bacteria and mold.
2. **Gaseous pollutants**. Chemicals derived from combustion processes are also found in gaseous form rather than in particulate form, as are products such as adhesives, paints, cleaning products, some pesticides, and fragrances.
3. **Liquids**. These chemicals are found in cleaning products, personal hygiene products, pesticides, etc.

The image below shows those chemicals present in your home that cause major health problems.

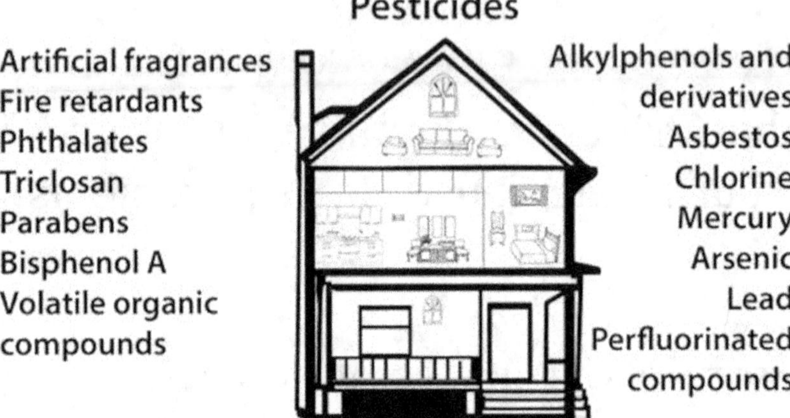

There is most likely a continuous, daily exposure to a "soup" of different chemicals in your home, which often causes headaches and allergic reactions (watery eyes, coughing, sore throat). Women, children and the elderly, are typically within the home for longer periods each day and tend to be most sensitive.

Most of us are usually outside our homes or in closed locations for no more than 10% to 20% of our time. Most people are aware of the pollution that exists outside, especially in large cities where we can sometimes see and even smell air contamination. The rest of the time we are usually indoors at home or in work places where we feel safe. What happens in these closed places where we spend most of our time? In reality, we live in a very polluted environment that we often cannot see. We are completely surrounded by chemicals that harm our body though we don't realize their potential damage. We ignore the pollution in our home where we are unknowingly exposed continuously to chemicals. As the air we breathe inside the house is usually not as pure as that outside air, it is vital to improve the quality of the air we breathe while inside, whether at home or at work.

According to a report by the U.S. Environmental Protection Agency (EPA), "indoor air pollution in homes, schools, offices and other buildings is one of the potential environmental risks to health, and is even more serious than imagined."

Exposure to these chemicals in the home can produce different effects on your health. As previously stated, they range from simple dizziness, nausea, allergic reactions, headaches, eye irritation, skin and throat problems like asthma or sore throat, to various cancers and occasionally death. The effects depend upon many factors including the type of the chemical, the mixtures of chemicals, your age, general health and genetic predisposition, and the duration of exposure.

What Toxic Chemicals are in Products in Your Home?

Here are some of the more toxic chemicals likely to be found in your home with a discussion of each.

Bisphenol A (BPA)

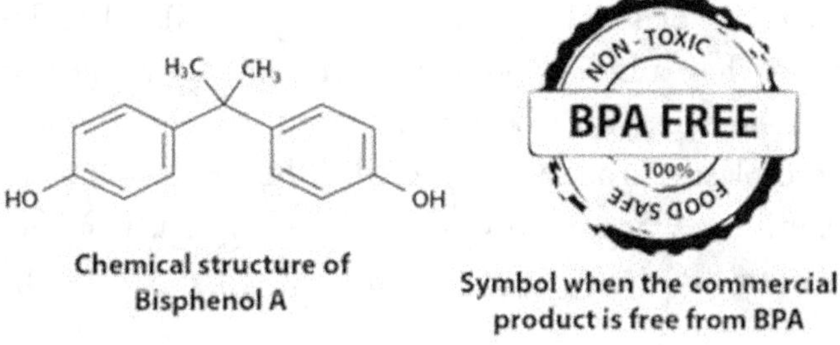

Chemical structure of
Bisphenol A

Symbol when the commercial
product is free from BPA

BPA was first synthesized in 1891 by the Russian chemist Aleksander Dianin. The chemical structure and biological action of BPA is similar to that of the human hormone, estrogen. Bisphenol A also strongly resembles the structures of DDT and PCB.

In the 1930s BPA was actually used by the medical community to replace the estrogen hormone. Later, diethylstilbestrol (DES), a similar but stronger chemical, came to be preferred over BPA. Years later, it was discovered that DES was highly toxic for pregnant women, skipping a generation and causing serious reproductive problems in females of the generation following those originally exposed to DES. Today, despite its chemical similarity to estrogen, BPA is used to make polycarbonate (a polymer of BPA), a hard, and clear plastic used in many consumer products. BPA is also found in epoxy resins, as a protective lining on the inside of certain metal-based cans used for foods and beverages. Note that the chemical structure of Bisphenol A (shown above) is extremely similar to that of DDT (see page 38).

Some plastic products that contain BPA include packaging for food and beverages such as water bottles, wine barrels, the underside of bottle caps, synthetic flooring materials, bottles for infants and babies, baby feeding cups, disposable cups, plastic cutlery, compact disks, eyeglass lenses, spare plastic parts for cars, paints, plastic water pipes, impact resistant safety equipment, medical devices (including plastic tubing and I.V. bags), fire-resistant materials, dental sealants and in some countries, even toys. BPA is also used in thermal paper receipts, stickers, fax paper, credit cards and manufactured plastic polyvinyl chloride (PVC). The United States produces more than a billion pounds of BPA annually, most of it used in plastic polycarbonates. It has been established that the BPA leaches out of most of these plastic products, especially when warmed, as for example with baby's milk or when microwaving food. This has resulted in significant increases in BPA found in human urine.[1]

The regulatory/safety issues surrounding BPA are exceedingly complex and controversial. But many individual states have imposed either a partial or a complete ban on its use in containers that come into contact with young children.[2] Exposure to BPA has been linked to diseases such as diabetes, breast and prostate cancers, infertility (low sperm count), uterine fibroids, endometriosis, (miscarriages) abortions, cardiovascular diseases, behavioral disorders including attention deficit hyperactivity disorder and obesity. Its association with all these illnesses is consistent with its classification as a known endocrine disruptor.[3, 4]

PHTHALATES

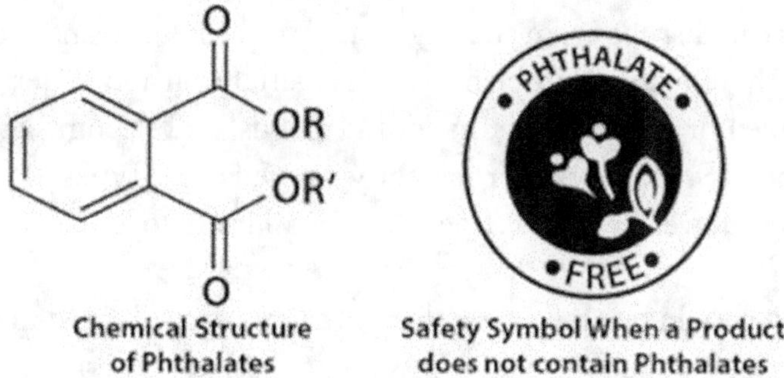

Chemical Structure
of Phthalates

Safety Symbol When a Product
does not contain Phthalates

Phthalates are a group of synthetic chemicals that are known endocrine disruptors. They are odorless, viscous liquids, used to soften various plastic materials. Plastic bottles that contain phthalates will be marked with a 03 recycling code number and should be avoided. Recycling numbers 2, 4, and 5 are considered the "safest" plastics; these plastics are the least likely to contain toxic chemicals.

Phthalates are used to soften and increase flexibility of the hundreds of popular plastics and vinyl polymers. When phthalates are added to plastics, the long polyvinyl molecules slide over each other, giving them the recognizable soft pliable nature of plastic products. Because they are not chemically bound to the plastic, the phthalates are continuously released from plastic products throughout their useful life, especially under elevated temperatures achieved when used in the microwave and when washing.

Phthalates are present in many PVC products, such as vinyl flooring coatings, soft toys made for babies and children, baby bottles, synthetic textiles, semi-synthetic glues and inks, and in solvents used in many cosmetics and personal hygiene products, including diapers.

Various studies have shown that phthalates are harmful to the male reproductive system.[3] They also cause damage to the liver and kidneys and may interfere with the production of the thyroid hormone, which plays an important role during brain development in fetuses and children.

Phthalates can disrupt brain activity related to the neurotransmitter dopamine, and thereby cause problems such as inattention and hyperactivity in children, memory impairment in adults, moods, and sleeping disabilities. In 2008 the U.S. Congress permanently banned three types of phthalates in any amount greater than 0.1 percent in children's toys.[5]

However, it should be made clear that phthalates are still used in hundreds of other products, such as vinyl flooring, adhesives, detergents, lubricating oils, automotive plastics, raincoats, and many personal-care products (such as soaps, shampoos, some toothpastes, hair sprays, and nail polishes). This continuous and pervasive use of phthalates is the reason for their continuing presence in the human body.[6, 7]

FLAME RETARDANTS

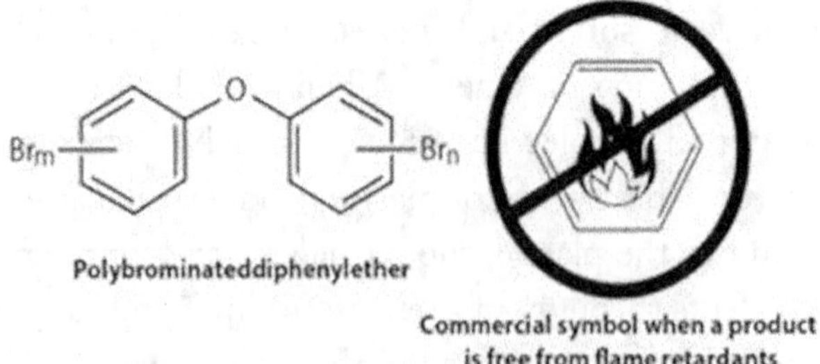

Commercial symbol when a product
is free from flame retardants

Flame retardants are a group of synthetic chemicals that share similar properties but have different structures. They are an example of the many chemicals whose consequences to the environment and human health, both in the medium and long term, were not studied at the time of manufacture and subsequent sale to the public.

The chemical structure similarities between the insecticide DDT, BPA, Triclosan, and the fire retardant organobromide are striking. One can speculate that the simultaneous presence of these various chemicals in a body have an additive deleterious impact on the same hormonal systems.

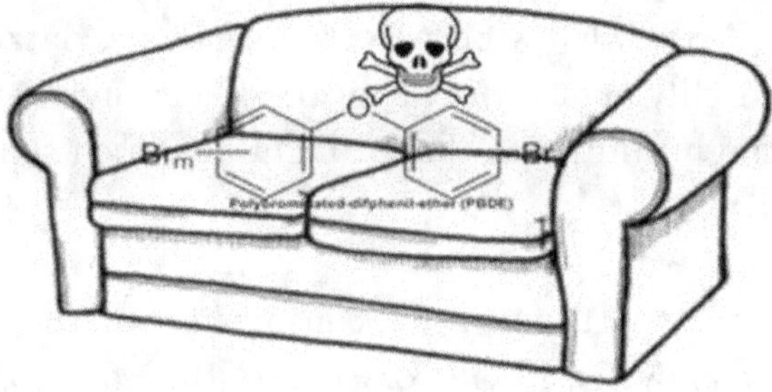

The industry adds these chemicals to almost all furniture items now on the market for the purpose of delaying or slowing combustion; yet it has been found that these chemicals often do not effectively serve this purpose. One of the more common fire retardants is the class called organobromides shown in the diagram above.

Use of flame retardant products is nothing new. Ancient Egyptians (450 BC) used aluminum sulfate and sulfur to reduce the flammability of treated wood. More recently, the Romans (200 BC) used aluminum sulfate and vinegar for the same purpose. The modern history of flame retardants began in the second half of the twentieth century with the development of synthetic polymers in the textile industry during World War II.

Many products in use today contain fire retardants. Plastics, textiles (fabrics, linens, pillows, some clothes, etc.), furniture for the home and office, some toys, kitchenware, coatings for electronics, hydraulic solvents to extract metals, defoamers, and sheeting over walls are some of the products that use synthetic polymers. Sadly, flame retardant chemicals are released from all these household items, enter the home environment and cause allergies and other illnesses especially in children and pets.

Because like BPA, these flame retardant materials are highly bioaccumulative in the body and are persistent (environmentally stable), they can be found almost anywhere in our environment, including freshwater sediments, fish and marine birds, in eggs, and even deep in the oceans and in Artic whales because the earth is contaminated with many of these highly persistent chemicals. Their environmental distribution is strikingly similar to that of DDT to which some are chemically very similar.

According to one report, when rats consumed minute amounts of the flame retardant known as TCP for 2 years they developed lesions in the ovaries and adrenal glands; male mice developed lesions in their liver. TCP also decreased fertility in rats and mice. Rats developed brain lesions.

There is not enough information available to determine with certainty whether phosphate ester flame retardants produce cancer in humans, but they are known to be highly neurotoxic, causing damage to the nervous system. After many legal battles, and thanks to the Toxic Furniture Right-to-Know bill, as of 2014 some consumers now have reasonable access to furniture made without toxic flame retardants. Unfortunately, this state bill applies only to sales in California and apparently does not extend to mattresses or other items. However, as of this writing, some 14 states have regulated or banned one or more fire retardants.[8]

PERFLUORINATED COMPOUNDS (PFCs)

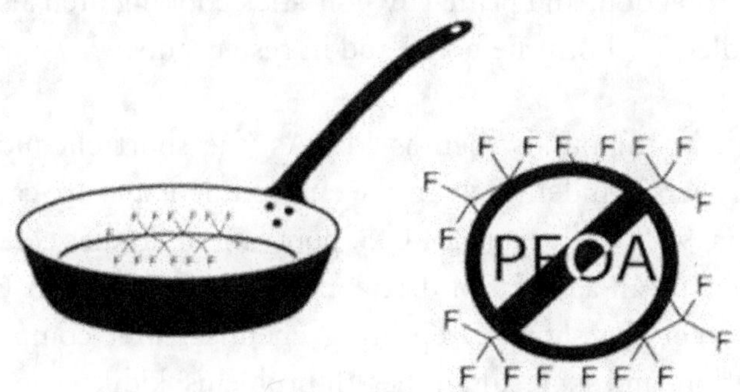

Perfluorinated compounds (PFCs) are a large group of manufactured chemicals that are made in long chains of repeating units called polymers. They are widely used to repel grease, stains, and water. PFCs may be used to keep food from sticking to cookware, to make sofas and carpets resistant to stains, to make clothes and mattresses more waterproof, and also appears in some food packaging, as well as in some firefighting materials. They are heat stable and resist chemical and biological decomposition.

PFOS and PFOA are cancer-causing chemicals that are persistent in the environment and bioaccumulative in the human body.[9]

One popular PFC is Teflon. Teflon (one of the longest chained synthetic polymers), has non-stick properties and is used to coat cooking utensils and cookware. Teflon was created in 1938 by Roy Plunkett, a chemist employed by the DuPont Company. DuPont decided to keep the existence of this substance secret while the company investigated its various potential uses.

In 1945 the DuPont Company named and registered the patent for Teflon. With virtually no government oversight, polymerized PFOA or Teflon has been used since the early 1950s in the manufacture of waterproofed clothing and hundreds of other industrial products such as cosmetics, textiles, non-stick and waterproof coatings, stain removers, cleaning products, plant protection, and primarily non-stick cooking utensils (pots, frying pans, ladles) for both the home and in restaurants.

Perfluorinated compounds such as PFOAs (the short chemical units of the polymer) persist indefinitely in the environment and are carried in the blood of some 98% of the general U.S. population. Studies concluded that there is probably an association between exposure to PFOA (not Teflon itself, but rather the shorter, repeating chemical unit components that make up Teflon) and six resultant health problems: kidney cancer, testicular cancer, ulcerative colitis, thyroid disease, hypercholesterolemia (high cholesterol), and pregnancy-induced high blood pressure.[10]

In other studies involving PFOA, additional adverse effects included altered lipid (fat) metabolism, a weakened immune system, and thyroid hormone level disturbances. Overheating of especially new pans coated with Teflon give off chemical fumes at high temperatures that typically result in short term nausea, and headaches in humans and more severe and deadly effects on birds.[11]

The potential cancer-causing capacity of PFOS and PFO is set out here.[12]

In research studies, the primary effects of exposure to PFOS and PFO found in rodents consisted of tumors in the liver, fertility issues, weakened immune systems, hormonal system disturbances and altered lipid metabolism.

PFCs, especially among them PFOA (also known as C8) and PFOS, are in the group of the many chemicals whose consequences to the environment and human health, both in the medium- and long-term, were apparently not known at the time of their first manufacture and sale. However, apparently Dupont, the manufacturer, knew that there was toxicity with C8 as far back as the 1950s.[12]

Over the decades, there has been disagreement and many controversial discussions regarding both the safety and long-term environmental persistence of PFOA and PFOS chemicals. DuPont has failed to report risk studies on C8 to the US EPA since 1981. Finally, in 2005 the EPA levied the highest ever financial penalty against a manufacturer for failing to submit such risk assessment data. DuPont refused to admit liability in the $16 million settlement and maintained they did not deliberately withhold information from the EPA.[13]

Some environmentalists believe that U.S regulators failed to exercise satisfactory safety oversight during the years that substances with C8 (PFOA) and PFOS and their so-called substitutes (wrapping paper, containers, etc) continued to receive approval for use in contact with food. In 2006, the EPA asked major chemical manufacturers, including DuPont and 3M, to set a goal of eliminating C8 from their products by January 31, 2015.[14,15]

In March 2014 the U.S. EPA designated PFOS and PFOA (C8) as emerging contaminants meaning chemicals with a perceived, potential, or real threat to human health or the environment.[16]

In animal research studies, some PFCs such as C8 – though apparently, not Teflon – disrupt normal endocrine activity and reduce immune function, cause adverse effects on multiple organs including the liver and pancreas, and cause developmental problems in rodent offspring exposed to them in the womb. Some progress has been made in reducing human PFC (C8) exposures since the phase out began in 2015.

Recent public information on the safety – or lack of safety – of the new next generation PFC-like substances in food contact substances, clothes, cosmetics, and cooking was at first largely non-existent. Now scientists have since learned that the new generation of PFCs may not be any safer.[17]

Sadly, PFCs are currently still being produced in Germany, Italy and at fifteen locations in China.[18]

VOLATILE ORGANIC COMPOUNDS (VOCs)

Volatile organic compounds (VOCs) originated with the development of the oil industry in the mid- nineteenth century with the appearance of gasoline in 1854. VOCs are one of the most common contaminants found in almost all of Earth's air. Exposure to these compounds occurs by inhaling contaminated air. Many VOCs are found in products like paints and lacquers, as well as moth repellents, air fresheners, hobby glue, wood preservatives, aerosol substances, caulking, and in many industries including the automotive industry and the dry-cleaning industry. VOCs are released into the atmosphere from all the aforementioned products, and can enter into the indoor air of homes and workplaces.

VOCs can cause irritation of the eyes and the respiratory tract, headaches, dizziness, visual disorders, fatigue, loss of coordination, allergic reactions of the skin, nausea, and memory disorders. Health effects from long-term exposures to VOCs can become even more serious, causing liver and kidney damage as well as diseases of the central nervous system. According to many research studies in toxicology, long-term exposure to VOCs by humans can be carcinogenic.

TRICLOSAN

Triclosan

Symbol on products
Triclosan free

Cl

DiChlorodiphenylTrichloroethane
(DDT)

Triclosan (a chlorinated compound, with a chemical structure strikingly similar to that of BPA) has a chemical structure similar to some of the most persistent toxic chemicals on earth, such as DDT. It is also closely related structurally to dioxin, and PCBs.

Triclosan, sometimes marketed under the name "Microban," is claimed to be a powerful antibacterial and antifungicidal agent. It was registered as a pesticide in 1969 and has been used by the cosmetic industry since 2001. In 2017, the U.S. Food and Drug Administration decided to ban the use of triclosan in certain household products such as soaps (but not in toothpaste) due to its lack of effectiveness as a microbial inhibitor; in fact, it actually selects and promotes antibiotic resistant bacteria. It is also active as an endocrine disruptor.[19] Triclosan is added to a variety of products because of its purported antibacterial action. It has a wide range of activity on bacteria the effectiveness of which is now being disputed.

Triclosan was originally used to control bacterial contamination on the hands, and hence was added to liquid dishwasher soaps, liquid hand soaps, mouthwashes, etc. Currently it is used in personal care products such as cosmetics, toothpaste, mouthwash, deodorants, anti-microbial cream products for acne treatment, lotions and soaps. Triclosan is also incorporated into a number of other popular consumer products, such as some kitchen utensils, toys, bedding, socks, and trash bags and is incorporated into plastics, textiles and medical device implants supposedly giving these materials antibacterial properties. It was also recommended to use triclosan-containing soaps on cooking and in cleaning cutting boards.

Triclosan has been detected as a contaminant in breast milk and fish, reflecting its inability to decompose in the environment and possible bioaccumulation much like BPA and DDT. Research studies correlate exposure to Triclosan with an increased risk of cancer. It can alter hormone regulation and interfere with fetal development by slowing it down.[20]

Triclosan is regulated in the U.S. and in the European Union. The U.S. FDA classifies it as a class III drug, while the Environmental Protection Agency, registers it as a pesticide, and considers it as a substance posing "high risk" to human health and the environment.

Artificial Fragrances

Musk Xylene (MX)
synthetic fragance

Artificial fragrances (synthetic ring based chemicals) are mostly endocrine disruptors with pleasant, persistent aromas. They first appeared in the late nineteenth century as an economic substitute for natural fragrances as they are cheaper and easy to synthesize. Some 90 natural fragrances are used only in the most expensive perfumes.

Today artificial (synthetic) fragrances such as the musk xylenes are added to many everyday products such as soaps, body creams, perfumes, cosmetics, and laundry detergents. Synthetic fragrances, also known as "synthetic musks," are often referred to as "nitro-musks" because of their chemical composition. Today synthetic fragrances are present in more than 5000 products on the market from personal care products and cosmetics to toiletries and household cleaners, air fresheners, perfumes, pesticides, and even to food and drink, as well as hundreds of other products for use in the home. The pleasant aroma of these synthetic fragrances motivates people to buy more commercial products.

The health problems caused by artificial fragrances or synthetic musks, was unknown until the1990s when it was discovered that they accumulate in the environment and deposit in the fatty tissue of living things. They are therefore persistent chemicals in the environment and bioaccumulative, much like DDT. The chance of a critical reaction triggering health problems is increased due to the fact that these musks are characterized by chemical stability and bioaccumulation in humans.

An examination of 17 commercial fragrances revealed that each one contained secret (unknown) chemical substances and also contained 4 or more endocrine disrupting chemicals.[21] Evidence of endocrine disruptor fragrance molecules have also been associated with various diseases in fish and amphibians. Since these fragrances volatilize and enter the air, technically they are also VOCs.

ALKYLPHENOLS AND THEIR DERIVATIVES (APS, APES)
The alkylphenols are a family of chemicals of different sizes and complexities. Alkylphenols (APs) are chemically modified to create surfactants, chemicals that increase the spreading and wetting ability of a solution, such as the even spreading of a dye through a material to

be stained. The chemical structure relationship between natural estrogen and 4-nonylphenol, which is a common surfactant used in the home, is striking. The diagram below shows the chemical makeup of human estrogen, 17-beta-estradiol (left) and 4-nonylphenol, surfactant precursor(right).

human estradiol (estrogen) surfactant precursor

The most widely used APEs are nonylphenol ethoxylates (NPEs) and, to a lesser extent, octylphenol ethoxylates (OPEs). Both are included in a list of known "persistent organic pollutants," or POPs. Alkylphenols have numerous unrelated commercial applications. They are used in the manufacture of antioxidants, lubricating oil additives, laundry and dish detergents, emulsifiers, paints, personal care products such as hair dyes and some plastics.[22]

Another alkylphenol, NPE, is considered to be an endocrine disruptor due to its ability to mimic the female hormone, estrogen, and in turn disrupt the natural balance of hormones.

Exposure to NPE is associated with the feminization of aquatic organisms, a decrease in male fertility, and shortened life spans of young fish. It is extremely toxic to other aquatic organisms as well. These chemicals persist in sediments where they can alter reproduction, induce feminization and hermaphrodism, and lower survival rates in salmon and other fish. Atienzar, (2002) et al describe the direct effects of nonylphenols and estrogen-inducing changes in both the function and structure of DNA of barnacle larvae, a mechanism that may be responsible for hormonal disruption effects described in other organisms.

Studies on APs and APEs have also revealed an association between exposures and problems such as leucoderma (localized pigmentation loss in the skin) and poor semen quality. Scientific studies have also linked them to an aberration in the timeline of sexual maturation.[23]

Blood tests have discovered a high percentage of APEs and their derivatives found in people living in many countries. Such a finding is concerning since these compounds have been associated with the above indicated health effects.

PARABENS

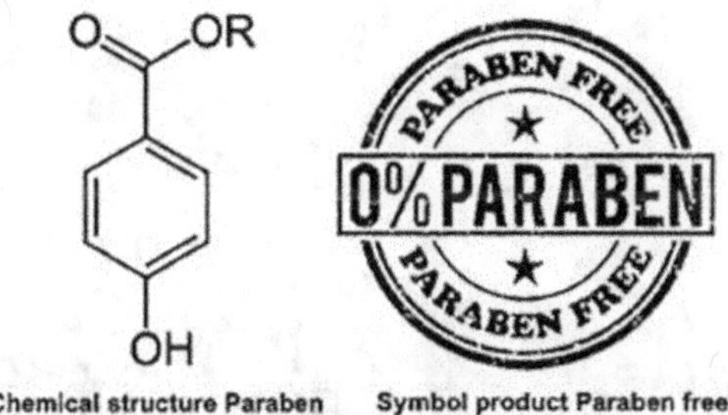

Chemical structure Paraben   Symbol product Paraben free

Parabens (chemically derived from the parent compound para-aminiobenzoic acid or PABA), are chemicals used primarily as preservatives in cosmetic products, pharmaceuticals and often in the food industry, because of their bactericidal and fungicidal properties. Methylparaben is more effective against molds, while propylparaben controls yeasts. Parabens may be found in toothpastes, deodorants, shampoos and cosmetics.

Natural parabens are found in some plants; for example, methylparaben is found in bilberry, where it acts as a natural antimicrobial agent. However, all parabens currently used in industry are of a synthetic origin.

When parabens are used in foods they are often partially decomposed and lose their foreign estrogenic activity. In experiments, parabens have been shown to bind to natural estrogen binding sites within cells but at much lower efficiencies than the natural estrogen hormone. Based upon the type of parabens found in breast tumors, researchers at the University of Reading in England believe it is possible that some parabens enter the body following skin contact from deodorants, creams, and sprays. PABA and parabens stimulate the growth of breast cancer cell lines in laboratory tests.[24]

Scientific studies have found these paraben chemicals to be associated with many diseases. Particularly disturbing was the finding that parabens are circulating in human blood at very low levels. As stated in this book (Chapter 2), endocrine disruptors are known to be active at miniscule concentrations (low parts per billion). PPB parabens are found in numerous locations in the home, and even in house dust.

SYNTHETIC PESTICIDES

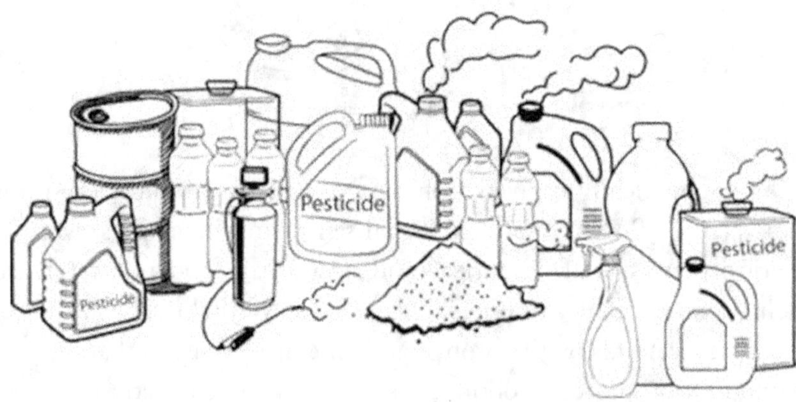

Synthetic pesticides pose several problems. Synthetic (man-made) pesticides pollute environmental water, and are responsible for the poisoning and death of domestic and farm animals, the death of fish in nearby waters polluted with the pesticide, and the death of other beneficial lifeforms like pollinators and other beneficial insects. Their most dangerous effect is human contamination sometimes causing serious illnesses to those exposed to them. Numerous pesticides are documented endocrine disruptors capable of causing environmental and human effects at ppb concentrations and less.[25]

Unfortunately, the use of synthetic pesticides has continually increased since World War II in both the number of pounds used and the number of registered active ingredients. The Environmental Protection Agency has now registered some 900 pesticide active ingredients formulated into some 20,000 pesticide products available for agriculture and home uses. Over 1 billion pounds of pesticides are sold annually in the United States.[26]

That 1 billion pounds amounts to about 3.5 pounds of pesticides sold for every man, woman, and child in the U.S. This 3.5 pounds per person represents more than *a billion times the level necessary to disrupt hormone activities.*

Some of the newer generation of insecticides, such as the neonicotinoids (neonics) are exceedingly toxic for honeybees making the discussion of the amount of pesticides used meaningless since a minute amount of these insecticides are lethal to honeybees. It is the toxicity of the ingredients that is most important, not only the amount used. For example 1 pound of neonics has the equivalent power of 10,000 pounds of DDT in killing honeybees.[27]

The scientific literature reveals that globally three million cases of human pesticide poisonings and 220,000 deaths occur each year.[25]

Although these manmade chemicals are intended to kill pests such as weeds, insects, fungi, rodents, algae, mites, and nematodes, their activity is not species specific. Thus, many other life forms including beneficial organisms that inhabit the earth are too often impacted by pesticide exposure – and we must include humans on this list.[28]

Recently, glyphosate, the active ingredient in the most commonly used weed killer, Roundup, has been added to that list of liver damaging pesticides. Incredibly, exposures to Roundup formulations in rats showed evidence of non-alcoholic fatty liver disease (NAFLD) at the minute concentration of 0.1 parts per billion (ppb) in drinking water fed over most of the life of the rats. The equivalent concentration of glyphosate in the sampled drinking water of these rats was 50 parts per trillion or some14,000 times *less* than the concentration allowed in U.S. drinking water.[29]

It is shocking that numerous food items contain glyphosate, ranging from about 1 to 1,000 ppb. This pesticide is commonly excreted in human breast milk and urine.[30,31]

The presence of glyphosate in human breast milk has been disputed by Monsanto and a scientist who has received grants from Monsanto. [32]

The World Health Organization's International Agency for Research on Cancer (IARC) recently designated glyphosate as "probably carcinogenic (cancer causing) to humans." It is the most commonly used weed killer in the world. The second most commonly used weed killer in American agriculture is called Atrazine, a known endocrine disruptor.

Very few pesticides have been tested for their hormone/endocrine disrupting activities, but among the 105 proven pesticide endocrine disruptors that have been tested, about 50% are found in insecticides, 21% are found in weed killers, and about 31% are present in fungicides.[25] You can find a list of 56 pesticides also believed to be endocrine disruptors here.[33]

That there is a huge medical impact resulting from the continued exposure of the human population to the billions of pounds of pesticides and other toxic chemicals in use, is a fact that cannot be disputed today because of all the published scientific studies.

The effects from all exposures to endocrine disruptors (not just pesticides), manifest in loss of IQ and intellectual ability, autism, attention-deficit hyperactivity disorder, obesity, diabetes, heart and vascular disorders, some cancers, cleft pallet and endometriosis. Scientists have estimated that the financial impact on human health (as stated in the Introduction) to be more than $300 billion per year in the United States alone as a result of medical expenses and lost wages. About 7,500 cases of intellectual disability in the U.S. each year, at an estimated cost of $44.7 billion have been attributed specifically to organophosphate insecticide exposures.[34]

Incredibly, there is no regulatory requirement in the U.S. that chemicals be studied for possible endocrine disruptor effects prior to their widespread availability for sale to consumers. The US EPA has been tasked with the job of developing methods to identify potential endocrine disrupting chemicals. However, very few chemicals (only 51 of the many thousands) have so far been analyzed during the nearly 20 years during which EPA scientists have been trying to optimize and develop new laboratory-based methods.[35]

As stated, there are some 20,000 pesticide formulations available to consumers. In separate analyses investigated largely by university scientists, some 85% of the 330 chemicals (including many pesticides) tested were found to be associated specifically with "non-alcoholic fatty liver disease (NAFLD).[36]

For Further Reading Chapter 3

1. https://www.hsph.harvard.edu/news/press-releases/bpa-chemical-plastics-leach-polycarbonate-drinking-bottles-humans/
2. http://www.ewg.org/search/site/bpa%20phaseout
3. https://en.wikipedia.org/wiki/Bisphenol_A#US_public_health_regulatory_history
4. http://www.packagingdigest.com/food-safety/history-bpa
5. http://www.national-toxic-encephalopathy-foundation.org/epafragban.pdf
6. http://www.medicaldaily.com/despite-federal-ban-phthalates-widespread-exposure-these-chemicals-still-exists-267079
7. http://www.cdc.gov/biomonitoring/phthalates_factsheet.html
8. https://www.stinson.com/Resources/Insights/2016_Insights/Flame_Retardants__A_Guide_to_Current_State_Regulations.aspx
9. http://www.ewg.org/kid-safe-chemicals-act-blog/2009/07/industry-calls-them-super-plastics-what-if-theyre-also-super-dangerous/
10. https://en.wikipedia.org/wiki/Perfluorooctanoic_acid#Toxicology_data
11. http://www.ewg.org/research/canaries-kitchen/teflon-kills-birds
12. https://theintercept.com/2015/08/20/teflon-toxin-dupont-slipped-past-epa/
13. http://www.washingtonpost.com/wp-dyn/content/article/2005/12/14/AR2005121402275.html
14. http://www.washingtonpost.com/wp-dyn/content/article/2006/01/25/AR2006012502041.html
15. http://www.ewg.org/research/teflon-chemical-harmful-at-smallest-doses/phased-out-still-threat
16. https://nepis.epa.gov/Exe/ZyNET.exe/P100LTG6.TXT?ZyActionD=ZyDocument&Client=EPA&Index=2011+Thru+2015&Docs=&Query=&Time=&EndTime=&SearchMethod=1&TocRestrict=

n&Toc=&TocEntry=&QField=&QFieldYear=&QFieldMonth=&QFieldDay=&IntQFieldOp=0&ExtQFieldOp=0&XmlQuery=&File=D%3A%5Czyfiles%5CIndex%20Data%5C11thru15%5CTxt%5C00000014%5CP100LTG6.txt&User=ANONYMOUS&Password=anonymous&SortMethod=h%7C-&MaximumDocuments=1&FuzzyDegree=0&ImageQuality=r75g8/r75g8/x150y150g16/i425&Display=hpfr&DefSeekPage=x&SearchBack=ZyActionL&Back=ZyActionS&BackDesc=Results%20page&MaximumPages=1&ZyEntry=1&SeekPage=x&ZyPURL

17. https://www.ewg.org/research/poisoned-legacy/how-safe-are-alternatives-long-chain-pfcs#.WfT6pmhSxPY

18. https://theintercept.com/2016/09/15/the-teflon-toxin-goes-to-china/

19. https://www.nrdc.org/stories/dirt-antibacterial-soaps

20. https://www.sciencedaily.com/releases/2014/09/140903121858.htm

21. http://www.ewg.org/research/not-so-sexy

22. http://www.toxipedia.org/display/toxipedia/Nonylphenol+and+Nonylphenol+Ethoxylates

23. http://www.hogarsintoxicos.org/en/riesgos/alkylphenols

24. http://www.webmd.com/breast-cancer/news/20151027/parabens-breast-cancer#1

25. https://www.ncbi.nlm.nih.gov/pmc/articles/PMC3138025/

26. https://www.ncbi.nlm.nih.gov/pmc/articles/PMC2946087/

27. http://www.takepart.com/article/2014/06/24/are-neonicotinoids-new-ddt-bees-and-other-wildlife

28. http://www.biologicaldiversity.org/publications/papers/SDLP_10Spring_Lopez.pdf

29. http://www.theecologist.org/News/news_analysis/2988500/roundup_residues_in_fo od_cause_fatty_liver_disease.html

30. http://www.glyphosate.news/2016-03-09-glyphosate-found-at-high-levels-in-mothers-breast-milk.html

31. https://www.omicsonline.org/open-access/detection-of-glyphosate-residues-in-animals-and-humans-2161-0525.1000210.pdf
32. https://www.forbes.com/sites/emilywillingham/2016/04/04/monsanto-linked-study-finds-no-monsanto-linked-herbicide-glyphosate-in-breast-milk/#1b98e19e24c0
33. http://www.beyondpesticides.org/assets/media/documents/gateway/health%20effects/endocrine%20cited.pdf
34. https://www.aacc.org/publications/cln/cln-stat/2016/november/17/endocrine-disruptors-cost-us-more-than-340-billion-in-health-and-other-costs
35. https://www.epa.gov/endocrine-disruption/endocrine-disruptor-screening-program-edsp-overview
36. http://ir.library.louisville.edu/cgi/viewcontent.cgi?article=1026&context=etd

How Do Chemicals Enter Your Body?

• • •

Chemicals enter your body in one of 4 ways:

* Through inhalation (airway or respiratory);
* Through your skin, mucous, membranes or eyes (topical);
* Through your mouth (oral and digestive);
* Through injection;

See the diagram.

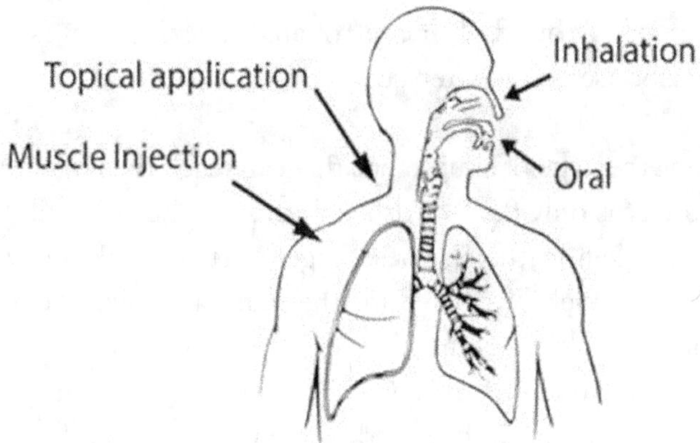

Exposure to potentially toxic chemicals present in numerous products and articles in the home allows for their entry into the body simultaneously by multiple pathways.

ENTRY BY INHALATION

This route allows entry of the exposed toxins into the body through the nose, mouth, larynx, lungs, bronchi, bronchioles and alveoli.

Inhalation is considered the primary route chemical contaminants found in the home and in the environment take to enter the human body. When you breathe in air, your body takes in all kinds of substances. Particles in the form of dust, and liquids that present as vapor and other gases mix directly with the air, which is contaminated by a toxic soup of chemicals. The many volatile chemicals that enter into our body by inhalation on a daily basis include fragranced products (air fresheners, candle fragrances, etc.), perfumes, detergents, pesticides, disinfectants, powders, and more. Any substance suspended in the atmosphere can be inhaled. Those particles of a certain size reach the deep lung's and are quickly and directly delivered into the blood stream. The average droplet size of a spray is initially 200-500 microns or about triple the size of a human hair.

Substances entering via inhalation can directly reach active receptors or "sites of action" within the respiratory system. Upon entry, these substances can cause a round of uncontrollable sneezing that is indicative of an allergic response and is often seen among children.

The average percentage of a substance that can reach the lungs when sprayed with an atomizer is only 0.2 %. Although this may seem small, the reader is reminded that when in the air these larger particles quickly evaporate and rapidly become smaller thus increasing the amount capable of entering deeply into the lungs. Droplets less than 7 microns can enter the air passages; only droplets less than 2 microns can enter the lung alveoli; droplets larger than 7 microns become trapped in the mouth, nasal passages, and the throat.

The total amount of a substance absorbed through the respiratory tract is a function of several factors: its concentration in the air, exposure time and the deepness and rate of inhalation. It is also important to consider the solubility of the aerosol substance in the moist environment of the respiratory system.

The ability to continually detect the same odors becomes less noticeable as our senses become "lazy" so to speak due to chronic exposures or with age. This loss over time of a sense of smell also increases the extent of potential respiratory exposures by inhalation so that we fail to notice this odor, and hence the length of exposure time required before detecting the toxic aerosol lengthens.

Additionally, these chemicals may also enter into the body via other routes as discussed below.

ENTRY THROUGH THE SKIN

The application of substances to the body surface (the skin), allows for chemicals to enter the body via a topical route. The skin is the largest organ of the body, with a total area of nearly 2 square meters and a mass representing some 12-15% of total body weight. It is made up of three distinct but very interrelated layers: the epidermis (the outermost), the dermis (large middle area) and the hypodermis or subcutaneous (deepest area) tissue.

The skin modulates body temperature, with thousands of nerve receptors that allow the sensations of heat, cold, and touch. Skin is distinguished by its color and texture. It reveals emotions through blushing when we are excessively nervous and perspiring when we are active. The skin protects the body from harmful substances in the environment. While it protects us by excluding microbes, there are many chemical substances that pass through it.

FACTORS THAT INFLUENCE ABSORPTION OF CHEMICALS BY THE SKIN

A number of factors increase the possibility that certain harmful chemicals may become absorbed through the skin and cause deleterious effects. These factors are chemical, environmental, anatomical, and physical factors.

CHEMICAL FACTORS

Some chemicals become diffused through fatty substances that surround skin cells and thus enter the body. Other chemicals enter via cell-to-cell permeation. A less usual path for entry is diffusion of the chemical through hair follicles and skin glands.

Many chemicals can penetrate the skin without adversely affecting it, yet move directly into the blood, and quickly distribute the contaminant or toxicant throughout the body.

When examining skin penetration we know that fat soluble chemicals are generally more readily absorbed and that substances that are both water soluble and contain fatty (lipid) components (like surfactants) readily cross the skin barrier to enter the body.

Of course, the chemical concentration, duration and frequency of exposure are also important.

ENVIRONMENTAL FACTORS

These consist of the following measures:

1. **Temperature:** An increase in the environmental temperature and humidity creating heat and sweat increase the ability of substances to be absorbed through the skin;
2. **Area of skin exposed:** The total area of skin contact that is exposed and the duration of the chemical exposure are important parameters that affect toxicant penetration;
3. **Increased chemical permeability:** Some substances (like solvents and detergents) cause damage to the components of the skin, thus decreasing the ability of the skin to act as an effective barrier and hence allowing increased absorption.

Physical and Anatomical Factors
These factors are as follows:

1. **Condition of the skin***:* Damaged skin (by scratches, cuts, burns or disease) is less resistant to chemical penetration than intact skin;
2. **Area of damaged skin:** Greater damaged skin surface areas provide more opportunities for a foreign chemical to enter the body.
3. **Skin thickness***:* When toxic substances come into contact with skin that is thin, the chemical arrives into the blood faster and this can cause more damage, and is thus more dangerous to one's health. The thinnest portion of the skin varies nearly 12-fold from the thickest portions of the skin. Skin over the male scrotum is the thinnest and is 11.8 times thinner than the area near the forearm, which is the thickest as shown in the diagram.

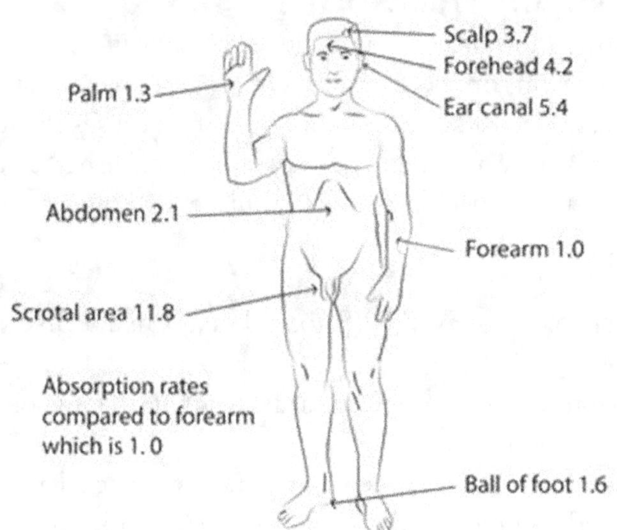

Those areas of the body with thicker skin can offer greater resistance to entry of toxic substances

Note that the higher the number the thinner the skin allowing absorption to occur more rapidly.

It is possible to avoid or eliminate penetration of topical chemicals into the body by washing the exposed area of skin quickly with water before the chemicals can enter into the body, or by using protective neutral creams when water is not available and by wearing suitable protective clothing before exposure.

There are two major types of poisonings when a chemical breaches the skin: local and systemic.

1. **Local poisoning:** Localized damage occurs when only the area that comes into contact with the toxic substance is affected.
2. **Systemic poisoning:** Systemic damage occurs when the damage extends beyond the area exposed creating damage throughout the body.

Entry Through the Mouth

Many of the toxic substances are introduced as food and beverages; thus we take in many toxins orally every day. Oral ingestion is a very common way chemicals enter the body. Oral ingestion often causes the most serious consequences since a liquid toxicant can become dispersed throughout the body via the throat, esophagus, stomach, and intestines.

The Two Categories of Acute (Short Term) Oral Poisoning

1. **Intentional:** Adults sometimes deliberately ingest poisons (suicides and homicides);
2. **Accidental:** Young children and others often accidentally ingest improperly stored toxic substances (often work related). When there is acute oral intoxication (AOI), the toxic substance has been consumed for one of the following reasons:

   Lack of proper hygiene
   You might eat or drink a product that has not been adequately washed, or handle or clean up a toxic chemical spill without

using suitable glove protection. This neglect is a common cause of poisoning by pesticides.

Contaminated food

Food can become contaminated during storage, transport, or when eaten beyond the recommended expiration date. Disease microorganisms can cause contamination as can storage of food in containers with toxic chemicals that may have leaked out onto the food.

Contamination can also be caused when products are mislabeled. This may happen when saving or repackaging food, water or other beverages in empty containers that had previously stored dangerous chemicals like pesticides or disinfectants or in "empty" containers that actually still contain chemical residue from a prior use. *Never reuse a container previously used to store chemicals; throw it way.*

Entry by Inoculation

The most direct entry of a substance into the body occurs through an accidental puncture, a new or pre-existing wound, by an animal bite (such as a snake bite), or by an insect bite or sting. These entries represent the most direct and quickest way that toxic chemicals can enter the blood and become distributed throughout the body. Harmful contaminating substances can also penetrate the body via a syringe or nozzle as when applying a tattoo.

Injecting a substance into the body with a syringe, may place the substance directly into a blood vessel, into muscle tissue, or shallower subcutaneous adipose tissue.

Direct injection into the blood stream causes a very rapid and direct effect. Injection under the skin or into muscle tissue, has a slower action, as the substance has to pass through several layers before reaching the blood vessels.

CHAPTER 5

Are There Non-Damaging "Safe" Levels of Exposure to Toxic Chemicals?

• • •

HARM FROM ALL CHEMICALS OCCURS at the cellular or molecular level. It is possible for even non-carcinogenic toxic chemicals to induce a serious illness or disease under certain circumstances. When a sufficiently large number of cells are damaged or die, the surrounding tissue(s) or organ(s) can be destroyed thereby causing serious or even fatal consequences.

NON-CARCINOGENIC SUBSTANCES

Usually, when only a few cells are damaged, the body is able to repair that damage and recover without any significant effect or consequence. In discussing non-carcinogenic substances, it is reasonable to believe that one can sustain some minimal damage which subsequently will lead to a complete recovery. The point of recovery and the extent of damage will vary depending on the age, general health, genetics, level of nutritional health and other factors of the individual exposed.

For non-carcinogenic chemicals, exposures considered to be "safe" can be estimated in a two-step process:

1. In the first step or stage of the process the highest dose causing no observable adverse effects in studies involving animals, tissue culture, or other biological assays is experimentally determined. This

dose level is designated as "No Observed Adverse Effect Level, or NOAEL (See the Figure below).

2. In the second stage, professional risk assessment analyses typically divide the NOAEL concentration level by a "margin of safety factor (MOS)." The MOS is used to reflect real world exposures with the goal to have a "margin of safety" in estimating the potential health effects of a given chemical. The MOS might also assist in "correcting" for possible synergy or continuous exposures to another chemical.

The chart below shows the correlation between the NOAEL and dose-response curve for a chemical, or, said another way, the toxicity of a chemical related to its dose and the extent of its effect in the biological investigative procedure.

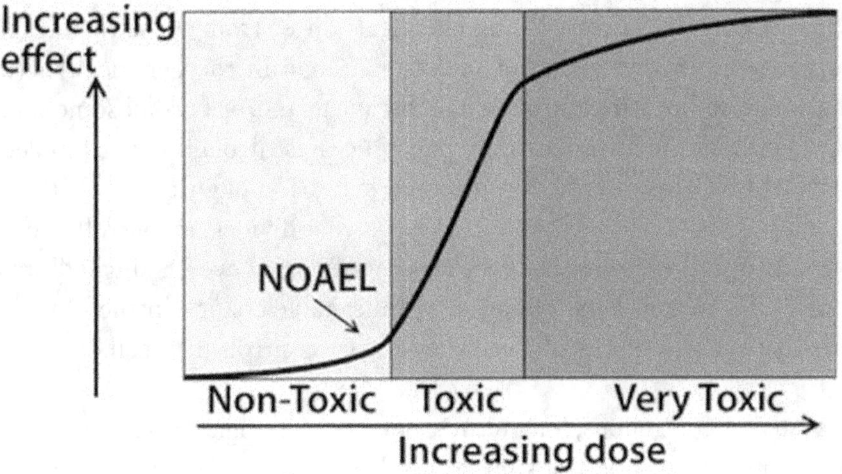

The greatest concentration that incorporates the margin of safety is thought to represent the "safe" degree of environmental exposure. If the chemical is a pesticide, test results from bioassays must consider both anticipated and actual levels of the chemical in food and water or in anything else in the real world before an allowable exposure level can be established.[1]

One problem here is that long after initial regulatory approvals are received, there may be some newly discovered adverse effects from the same chemical in the future. An example of this is the current recognition that lead is more harmful at lower concentrations than was previously believed. The EPA is required to only reexamine tolerance levels of a chemical after every 15 years in commerce; thus, safety cannot be guaranteed by the registration of any chemical by a federal regulatory agency.[2]

The reasons there are differences in the potency of toxic chemicals are not always well understood; it may be due to the ease by which different chemicals enter the cell and access the genetic material, or with how chemically reactive the particular substance is.

CANCER-CAUSING CHEMICALS

Carcinogenic or cancer-causing chemicals differ from those that are not carcinogenic in that they can induce a change in the genetic structure of a single cell causing chromosome breakage and/or chromosome mutation. Without effective natural repair processes through normal molecular reactions, this altered chromosome may be enough to ignite a chain of continuous reactions that lead to a cell that divides uncontrollably and expands into other tissues. This can happen with even a single "hit" or contact if a certain gene mutation or inheritable change in the DNA occurs that causes the loss of a cell's regulatory controls over cell division.

Repeated or continuous, long term exposures to a single toxicant conducted under laboratory conditions might result in a loss of control over cell division when the initial mutation(s) cannot be repaired by normal molecular reactions. When intact animals, including humans, become exposed at similar concentrations, the reaction may or may not cause detectable harm simply because of differences in complexities of laboratory tissue cultures as compared to whole animal exposures. Carcinogens may differ among themselves in potency, meaning, how likely they are to cause cancer given specific exposures. For example the fungal toxin called Aflatoxin B is a million times more powerful than trichloroethylene and much more likely to cause cancer. Dioxins are considered to be the most toxic cancer-causing chemicals known.[3] Formaldehyde is also generally believed to cause cancer but requires more continuous or longer term exposures and rates of cancer are low. Shorter term exposures to formaldehyde induce nausea, wheezing, eye irritations, etc, but apparently there is little cancer risk.[4]

ENDOCRINE DISRUPTING CHEMICALS

There are at least two novel properties associated with exposures to endocrine disruptors. First, as stated earlier, endocrine disruptors are active in causing medical issues at extremely low concentrations, some one-thousand to one-million times below that of effects seen with many other toxic chemicals. The very low concentrations of action can mislead many to believing there is no danger. The second unique issue associated with EDs is that the dose response curve as indicated earlier in calculating the NOAEL level, is much more complex. Technically, the dose response curve is referred to as non-monotonic. This means an effect from an ED may be greater at very low concentrations than at intermediate levels. This confounds the age-old theory about toxic chemicals profoundly stated in the 15th century by Paracelsus, "the dose makes the poison." Paracelsus meant that higher doses of chemicals are more serious than lower doses. This does **not** apply to endocrine disruptors. Little did Paracelsus know that the minuscule dose of EDs could be so effective a poison.

Because of all these variable characteristics with different toxic chemicals, one realizes how laboratory tests that only use one chemical or a onetime exposure to a chemical to investigate toxicity can lead to highly artificial outcomes. Often such laboratory tests do not reflect real world conditions. The reasons for the differences in potencies among toxic chemicals are not always well understood, but may be due to the ease with which different chemicals enter the cell and access the genetic material, or how chemically reactive the substance is blocking or stimulating a cell reaction.

For Further Reading Chapter 5

1. https://www.epa.gov/pesticide-tolerances/about-pesticide-tolerances
2. https://www.epa.gov/safepestcontrol/food-and-pesticides
3. http://www.ejnet.org/dioxin/.
4. https://www.cancer.gov/about-cancer/causes-prevention/risk/substances/formaldehyde/formaldehyde-fact-sheet

CHAPTER 6

How Do Endocrine Disruptors Work?

• • •

DEFINING PRECISE MECHANISMS OF HORMONE interference activities by endocrine disruptors has been difficult. However, some mechanisms of action including hormone substitution, blockage or alteration of hormonal levels have been described. These modes of interference typically occur when an endocrine disruptor has a chemical structure similar to the natural hormone. This can have one of the following consequences:

1. **Endocrine disruptors like DDT, PCBs, PPBs, and some plant estrogens** mimic or imitate the action of natural hormones confusing, for example, cellular estrogen receptors that develop or maintain female characteristics. Such reactions have the potential to slow or block the natural reactions and impact sexual and reproductive functions.

2. **Androgen antagonists** (also called androgen disruptors) counteract the effects of the natural male sex hormones testosterone and dihydrotestosterone by binding to the male hormone receptors. Included among the long list of androgen disruptors are Bisphenol A, phthalates, trichlosan and DDE (DDT breakdown product), and PCBs. Side effects of androgen disruptors in men include breast development, general feminization, hot flashes, sexual dysfunction, infertility, and osteoporosis. Certain androgen endocrine disruptors are medically prescribed to treat

prostate cancer, acne, and precocious puberty. The fungicide Vinclozolin (used on fruits, vegetables, ornamental plants, and turf grass) can mimic male hormones and has androgen disruptor activity.

3. **Some EDCs** act by modifying the synthesis and metabolism of natural hormones, or modulating or interfering with physiological levels, either by raising or lowering their concentrations. This is the case of phytoestrogens (flavones, isoflavones, cumestans, lignins) and mycoestrogens (produced by fungi) that induce the appearance of mammary glands in male mammals.

The three images that follow show the relationship of the hormone to the cellular receptor.

The Normal Reaction

In a normal situation, the normal amount of the hormone binds to the cellular receptor and triggers a reaction:

1. Normal

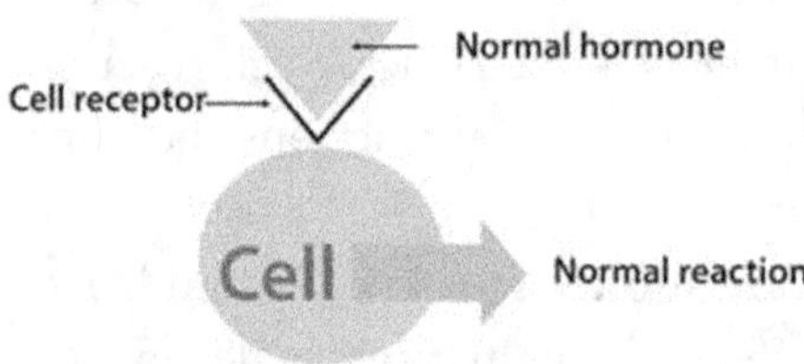

When a cell binds with an endocrine disrupting chemical, one of several consequences are possible in the reaction:

THE BLOCKED REACTION:

Endocrine disruptors can resemble the natural hormone chemically, mimic it and bind tightly to the receptor thus interfering with the reaction by blocking it.

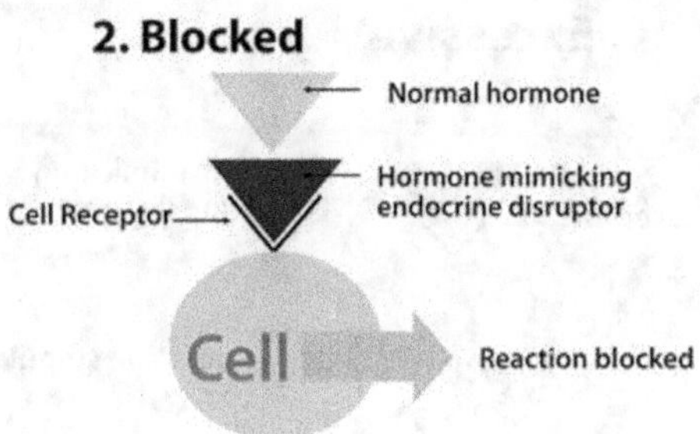

THE INSUFFICIENT REACTION

Endocrine disruptors can bind to the cellular receptor and generate a weaker reaction than normal and/or at the wrong time. This happens because of an imperfect match in chemical structures between the cell receptor and the endocrine disruptor.

The Excessive Reaction

Endocrine disruptors can bind to the cellular receptor and generate a more potent reaction at normal and/or at the wrong time in a cellular or developmental process.

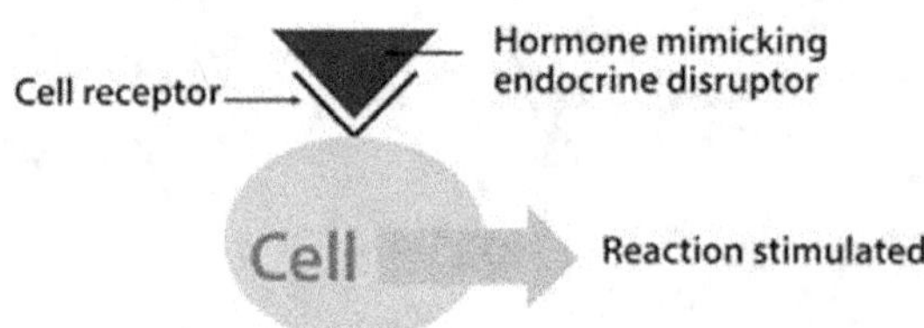

Natural hormones are normally produced at very low levels since there are very few receptor targets in each cell. This is why toxic external chemical substances (endocrine disruptors) can produce adverse effects on the animal or human endocrine system even if the doses are far too low to show the least possible immediate toxic response. Endocrine disruptors work at levels of parts per billion and even parts per trillion.

CHAPTER 7

Does it Matter?

...

ARE YOU ESPECIALLY VULNERABLE TO DANGERS FROM CHEMICALS?

TOXIC CHEMICALS IN THE HOME (or workplace) can affect anyone; however, there are groups that are particularly vulnerable and include young children, pregnant women the fetus, and older people.

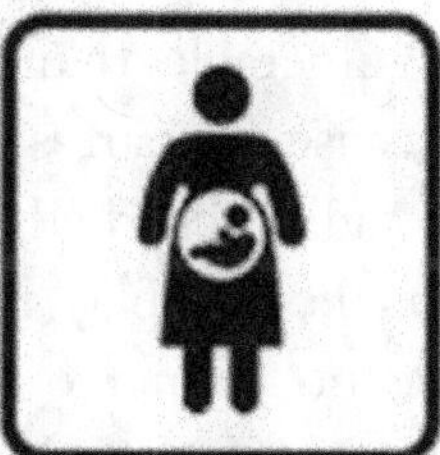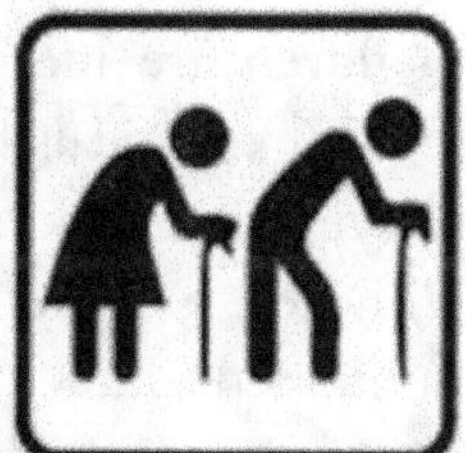

YOUNG CHILDREN

Young children are especially susceptible to the effects of chemicals in their environment as they easily accumulate in their body. There are probably more exposure opportunities, and children's natural resistance mechanisms are not yet fully developed. In some instances, the exposure to chemicals during childhood can cause serious health damage that may only become obvious much later in life.

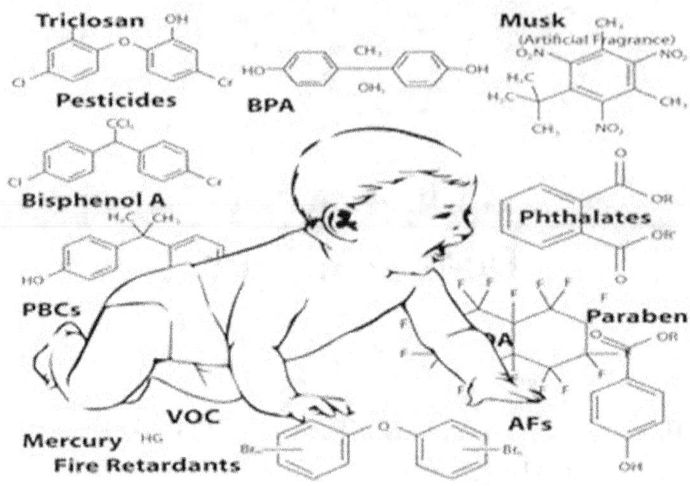

Factors Contributing to the Poisoning of Young Children

1. Children are more vulnerable than adults to the harmful effects of chemicals because they are still growing and developing. Chemicals are more readily absorbed into growing tissues.

2. Children have a tendency to play in places that may be contaminated. They are too young to understand proper hygiene measures and avoid unsafe situations. Inappropriate parental oversight also contributes to their unnecessary and unhealthy exposures.

3. Children breathe more rapidly than adults and also are closer to the ground. As such, their exposure to volatile organic compounds (VOCs), fire retardants and other harmful chemicals is greater in addition to being exposed to diverse substances present in house dust, which can be ingested directly through hand- to-mouth transfers.

4. The skin of children is more permeable and they eat and drink more in proportion to adults which facilitates incorporation of pollutants into their body.

5. Their organ systems that act to eliminate increased amounts of toxic chemicals to which they may be continuously exposed (such as the liver) are not yet fully matured.
6. Children cannot read or understand labels.

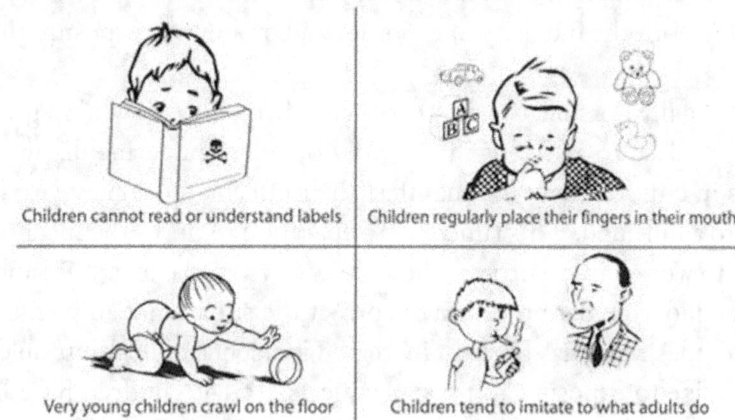

7. Children regularly place their fingers in their mouth and sometimes in their nose and ears all of which facilitate entry of toxic chemicals into the body;
8. Very young children crawl on the floor, which gives them access to dangerous products that may not be visible to adults;
9. Children tend to imitate what adults do;
10. Children do not understand the consequences of eating or drinking something that is potentially harmful.

SOURCES OF THE MOST COMMON CHEMICAL POISONINGS IN CHILDREN:

1. Medicines and drugs;
2. Rodent and insect poisons;
3. Cleansers (liquid and powder);
4. Personal hygiene products.

The Child's Room

Perhaps surprisingly, reports indicate that the child's room can be one of the most harmful places in the house. It might contain many endocrine disruptor products harmful to the child's health. The child's room may also have less space than other rooms in the house and poor air circulation thus increasing both the intensity of exposure and prolonging exposure time.

It is not usually possible to know precisely where, how, or when a given exposure will lead to a serious illness. Additionally, endocrine disruptor exposures in children may not manifest their effects until many years later, even into adulthood. This time/space separation removes the incentive for parents to work hard to protect their children from the mysteries and miseries of endocrine disruptors or to correct the situation. Sadly, in the last three decades there has been an increased incidence of health problems in children due to exposure to toxic chemicals. Today, children have higher incidences of allergies, childhood asthma, as well as many types of cancers and neurological disorders.

Childhood Asthma

Exposures to volatile organic compounds (VOCs) can significantly increase the risks of developing asthma. Solvents, the adhesives for floors, paints, cleaning products, waxes and polishes, air fresheners and fragrances, painted or varnished furniture and plastic toys expose children to these VOCs.[1]

Investigation has revealed that domestic exposure to volatile organic compounds, even when below those limits declared as "safe", may significantly increase the risk of childhood asthma.

Infant cancers

New studies associate leukemia (blood cancer) in children with exposure to substances such as household pesticides. Other studies associate these substances with brain cancers.[2]

Studies have also associated the use of flea and tick products, termite control products, anti-lice shampoo and pesticides in the house or garden, with these childhood diseases. Flea collars contain hormone disrupting chemicals as do pesticides often used on farms (pyrethroids and weed killers, other insecticides). Children become exposed through close association with their pets.[3]

Other studies have found that pesticides used for lawn care, result in a significant increase in the risk that a child may suffer medulloblastoma (a type of brain cancer).[4]

Neurological disorders in children

Researchers at Harvard and Mt. Sinai Medical School have described the harmful effects that chemicals such as lead, household industrial chemicals (solvents), and pesticides (DDT, chlorpyrifos) have on the development of the brain in children.[5]

Lead, once common in paints and water pipes (and still present in some 10 million water services in American homes), has been directly associated with many cases of mild childhood mental retardation (loss of I.Q.), kidney problems, developmental problems, attention deficit disorder, hyperactivity and irritability, and even alterations of the brain associated with impulse control.

Lead has also been associated with a very significant increase in aggressive and violent behavior by children, and even later criminal behavior in children with certain levels of lead in their bodies. Besides lead, other pollutants can also affect infant neurological development. Contaminants that may be associated with attention deficit disorder and hyperactivity are all too common in our lives. They include manganese, VOC solvents, PCBs, cadmium, pesticides such as pyrethroids, organophosphates, diazinon, chemicals like PBDE, trichloroethylene, and others, many of which are contained in pesticide formulations for home and garden use and in commercial formulations for spraying fruit and killing of mosquitoes. Studies show that residues of pesticides such as organophosphates, and pyrethroids used to combat mosquitoes, present even at very low concentrations of food (such as those typically found in products for sale and considered many times below the legal limits) can have detrimental effects on the brain of children including an association with ADHD in boys and are estrogen mimics.[6]

Similar problems have been associated with exposure to pollutants other than pesticides. Dioxins, furans, and other industrial contaminants may reach children when present in beef and swine, fish, and dairy products. The diagram below shows the routes that common chemicals in the home travel to reach the fetus when the mother is exposed during pregnancy.

PREGNANCY AND THE FETUS

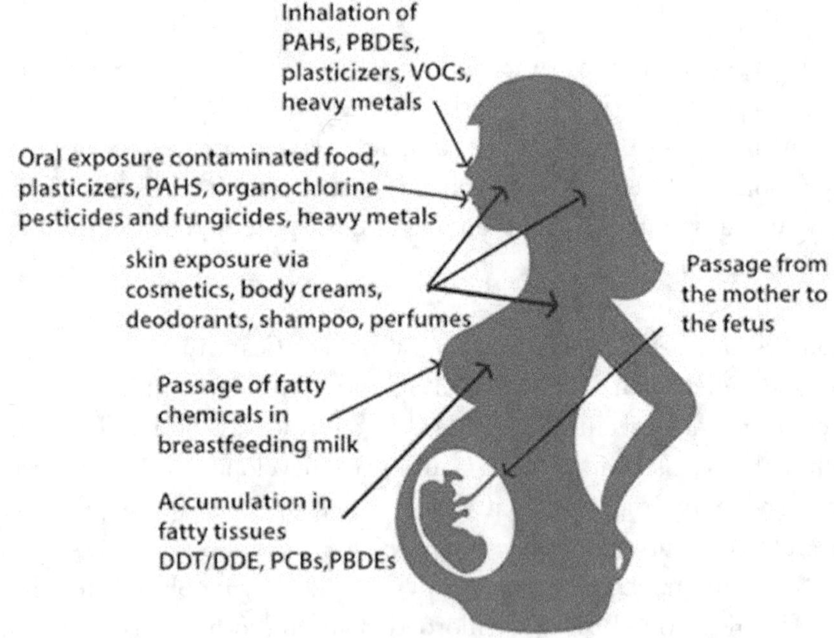

During its first trimester, the fetus is especially susceptible to even very low levels of toxic chemicals. The fetus is undergoing rapid differentiation; the development of organ systems, especially the brain, is far from fully developed and there are few protective mechanisms in place. Any interference that disturbs the natural processes, including the quantity and diversity of hormones that reach the fetus, is likely to have profound effects with life-long consequences. Some chemical-associated problems may manifest in spontaneous abortions (miscarriages), premature births and/or birth defects, loss of I.Q., and other issues.

The following syndromes and illnesses have been associated with fetal exposures to toxic chemicals: Premature birth, congenital malformations at birth including congenital heart defects and malformations of the reproductive system, defects and malformations of the central nervous system including decreased I.Q., skeletal malformations, cleft lip and cleft palate.

Problems also may develop later in childhood, such as neurodevelopmental damage or childhood cancers and even diseases that manifest decades later as adults, such as cancers and cardiovascular problems.

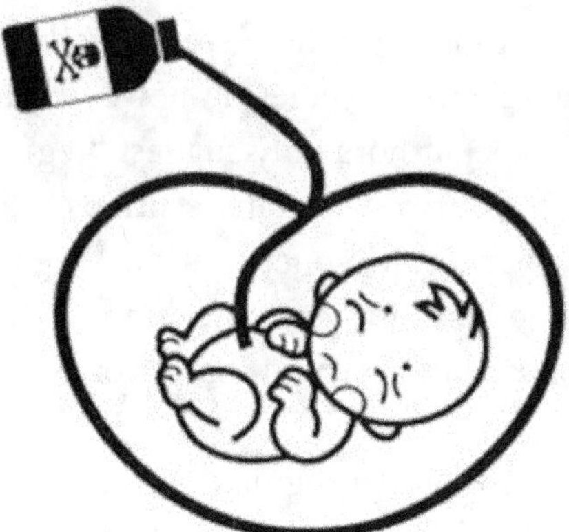

It is troubling that numerous toxic chemicals have been found within the bodies of pregnant women. A study published in 2009 by the Environmental

Working Group in Washington, D.C. found over 200 chemicals present in the umbilical cord blood of 10 babies.[7]

A 2011study found some 163 chemicals present in some 268 pregnant women. Certain polychlorinated biphenyls (PCBs), organochlorine pesticides, perfluorocarbons, phenols, PBDEs, phthalates, polycyclic aromatic hydrocarbons, and perchlorate were detected in nearly all the women.[8] It was further observed that some mothers tested positive for having several contaminants simultaneously in their blood that could target the same organ or biochemical process of the fetus, such as perchlorate, PCBs, PBDEs, and triclosan. All of these can affect maternal thyroid hormones, and go on to affect development of the reproductive system in their male children. Toxic substances are passed from the mother to the fetus through the amniotic liquid.

It is very easy to demonstrate, as I have in this book, that there are numerous exposures to these chemicals in our everyday lives. "Full time stay at home" pregnant women are continually exposed to many of these toxic chemicals. There are some statistically validated studies that relate exposure to specific chemicals to the illnesses indicated above. However, there is little published information to tell us with certainty whether the more subtle and prolonged exposures at home specifically correlate with any of these diseases. Many scientific studies do however, show a suggestive relationship although some authors only suggest "regulatory caution" until such relationships are confirmed.[9] This cautious regulatory perspective in my opinion, derives from the concept of the "silent" epidemic between exposures to endocrine disrupting chemicals and a disease presence when the illnesses are separated in time and space from specific exposures.

There is a failure in America to regulate on the basis of the precautionary principle. The World Health Organization published a report about the precautionary principle and why today's highly technological developments with chemicals demand more and more precautionary considerations prior to exposing the public to new products that have not been thoroughly studied as to their toxicity. The approach of this WHO study, in part, declared the following "... *precautionary actions ultimately aim at continuously reducing and if possible removing exposures to potentially harmful substances, activities and other conditions. If progress is to be made in this direction, one should encourage the replacement of dangerous substances and activities with less dangerous substances or technologies where suitable alternatives are available.*"

CHEMICALS ASSOCIATED WITH FETAL DISORDERS

The problems that exposure to chemicals reek on the general populace have been discussed to some extent above. Unfortunately, there is a host of disorders that have been linked to newborns. Most of these toxic substances found in the home have been clearly linked to numerous and relatively common problems at birth as for example, fetotoxicity miscarriages, birth defects, premature birth, low birth weight, and developmental disorders of the brain or the reproductive system, among other problems.[10]

Exposure to phthalates has been linked to incidents of male babies expressing feminization or less than complete virility. The use of pesticides in the home during pregnancy has been associated with an increased risk of leukemia and non-Hodgkin lymphoma in the baby's later life. The frequency or exposure in the use of some pesticides during pregnancy, specifically pyrethroids, has also been linked by some studies to a significant drop in the rate of mental development of children born to mothers exposed to this pesticide three years after birth. Similarly, residues of organophosphate pesticides found in the mother, has been associated with effects on the brain development of children.

Certain fresheners or fragrances used in the home have been found to cause children under six months old to experience an increased number of earaches and diarrhea as well as being linked by some studies to an increased risk of headaches and postpartum depression in women who remained in homes where these products were used daily.

Other research shows an association between the use of chemicals in the home during pregnancy and childhood asthma at birth. In one study, it was determined that those pregnant women who often used products such as disinfectants, bleach, carpet cleaner, window cleaner, liquid dry-cleaning solutions, aerosols, air fresheners (spray, stick, and aerosol), turpentine/paint thinner, paint remover, paint, varnish or pesticides/insecticides, and a host of other products, had a higher risk of asthmatic children than those who made less use of these products. Scientists have reached the conclusion that the cause of the asthma could be prenatal exposure and/or the effect of subsequent exposure in the early stages of life.

Although much research has been done concerning risks from the use of chemicals in the home during pregnancy and the first months of life of the newborn, the problem is that many pregnant women lack the information. Prenatal exposures to various toxic chemicals and their specific adverse health effects are clearly summarized in this brief article by "Physicians for Social Responsibility". Surely pediatricians, on the front line of caring for infants, will know more about causal relationships between endocrine disruptors and diseases than regulators.[11]

What Other Chemicals Are Toxic for the Fetus?

The chemicals associated with these maladies include, but are not limited to: formaldehyde, various petroleum-based solvents, glycol ethers, trichloroethylene, tetrachloroethylene (used for dry cleaning and probably carcinogenic), toluene, xylene, ethylene oxide, trichloroethane, arsenic, Bisphenol A, trihalomethane products, chloroform, some fungicides, lead, mercury, methylene chloride, thiazine's (ring compounds used to make dyes and insecticides), soot, exposure to endocrine disruptors such as benzene, DDT /DDE, ethylene oxide, lead, phthalates, and phenoxy herbicides like 2,4-D, PCBs, pentachlorophenol.

THE ELDERLY

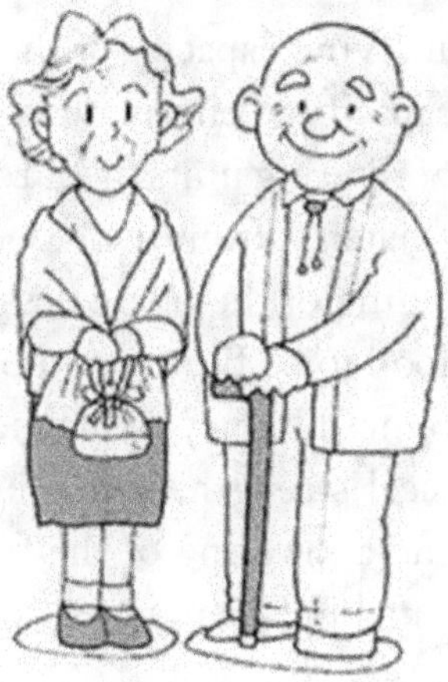

Older people are at risk of chemical poisoning in the home for several reasons. Primary among them is the fact that over the years our body undergoes many changes.

The bones, muscles, eyes, hearing, etc. suffer a physiological evolution, better known as "aging," which causes changes in the functions of each of the body's organs and systems. Some changes that take place in the human body over the years:

1. Changes in the mass of the organs and bones.
2. Changes in pharmacodynamics (that is, how drugs affect the body).
3. Changes in the autonomic nervous system (body functions not consciously directed like heartbeat, digestion, respiratory rate, pupillary response, urination, and sexual arousal).
4. Psychological changes.
5. Endocrine changes (changes in hormone levels).
6. Pulmonary (lung) changes.
7. Cardiovascular changes.

8. Global functional changes (characterized by impairment of daily living activities).
9. Changes in the purifying capacity of the liver and kidneys resulting in decreased capacity to eliminate toxins from the body:
    * The number of filtering units (nephrons) in the kidneys, which remove waste material from the blood, is reduced.
    * There is hardening of the blood vessels supplying the kidney, causing the blood to be filtered more slowly.
    * The total amount of kidney tissue mass is reduced.
10. A decline in physical strength, the level of the body's ability to fight off disease and a lowering of the functional efficiency of all body organs, thus making them more vulnerable to damage.

CHALLENGES FACED BY THE ELDERLY THAT CAN LEAD TO DRUG INTOXICATION

1. Most seniors have vision problems and sometimes have difficulty reading labels even with glasses.
2. Medications of similar colors and pill shapes tend to be confusing.
3. Older adults often take several medicines on a daily basis, often at different times of the day; it becomes easy to forget or duplicate a medication.
4. Some older adults have medical conditions that cause confusion.
5. Many seniors live alone and do not have adequate reminders to take a medication or to duplicate a medication.
6. Taking different medications daily, as is common in the elderly, can result in unwelcome interactions, such as diminishing the beneficial effects (becoming less effective) or potentiating side effects. Under these conditions it is essential to have a trusted pharmacist.

The problems above associated with drug intoxication can occur as early as 60 years of age. But when over 85 years of age, mistakes in taking drugs can impact 25-50% of elderly people. As the elderly are more fragile than younger people, a given exposure to a toxic chemical can produce more serious complications.

It is not uncommon for drug intoxication to go unnoticed or undervalued in the elderly and hence not recorded, especially when they live alone. National toxicology information centers indicate that accidental chemical intoxications are the third leading cause of death among people 65 years of age and older and account for nearly 5% of all types of injuries in older people.

Like children, older people have a high risk of having an accident in their own home. Falls, bumps, burns, poisonings and other events are the most prevalent types of accidents.

CAUSES OF MOST COMMON HEALTH ISSUES IN THE ELDERLY

* Exposures to toxic chemicals in and around the home.
* Errors with medications.
* Abuse or misuse of medicines.
* Misuse of personal and household hygiene products.
* Exposure to carbon monoxide.
* Animal and insect bites or stings.
* Attempted suicides.

For Further Reading Chapter 7

1. https://marylandpirg.org/blogs/blog/mdp/testimony-green-cleaning-supplies
2. https://www.hsph.harvard.edu/news/hsph-in-the-news/pesticide-exposure-in-childhood-linked-to-cancer/
3. https://well.blogs.nytimes.com/2015/09/21/pesticides-tied-to-childhood-cancers/
4. https://www.ncbi.nlm.nih.gov/pmc/articles/PMC2688447/
5. http://www.medicalnewstoday.com/articles/272633.php
6. https://www.cincinnatichildrens.org/news/release/2015/study-links-pesticide-ADHD-in-boys-06-01-2015
6. https://www.scientificamerican.com/article/newborn-babies-chemicals-exposure-bpa/
8. https://www.ncbi.nlm.nih.gov/pmc/articles/PMC3114826/
9. http://www.sciencedirect.com/science/article/pii/S0378427413013659
10. https://en.wikipedia.org/wiki/Environmental_toxicants_and_fetal_development
11. http://www.psr.org/assets/pdfs/prenatal-exposure-to-chemicals.pdf

CHAPTER 8

Twenty-Six Ways to Reduce The Dangers of Chemicals In Your Home

• • •

WHILE IT IS PRACTICALLY IMPOSSIBLE to remain free of all products containing potentially hazardous chemicals, exposures can be reduced by keeping some basic principles in mind.

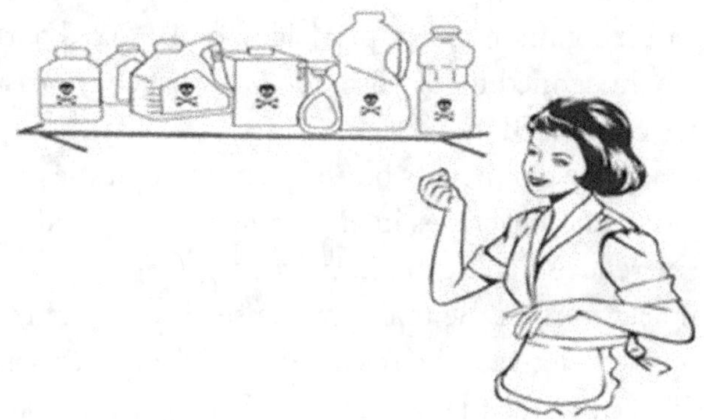

1. Choose products that are "free" from the chemicals mentioned above to avoid having them as "house guests" that end up polluting.
2. Always read the instructions before using or having contact with a commercial product.
3. Minimize the use of cosmetic and personal hygiene products with dangerous chemicals, especially before and during pregnancy.

4. Become familiar with chemicals linked to hormonal disorders and always read labels.
5. Keep chemicals in their original bottles or containers.
6. Avoid mixing chemicals such as ammonia and bleach, pesticides, disinfectants, etc., because they can create mixtures even more dangerous to your health and your family.
7. If you must use pesticides or other chemicals around the home, wear protective clothing (gloves, long sleeves, long pants, socks, shoes) as appropriate.
8. Do not use food containers such as cups, empty water bottles, or empty food jars to store chemicals, such as cleaning solutions, pesticides, or beauty products.
9. Open windows or turn on the exhaust fan when using chemicals such as household detergents, disinfectants, household cleaners, pesticides.
10. Eat whole foods, especially fresh ones. Processed and packaged foods are a common source pesticides, of BPA, and phthalates particularly in canned foods; also, foods packaged in plastic containers may contain BPA.
11. Buy products sold in glass bottles instead of plastic or cans.
12. Store food and beverages in glass containers instead of plastic and avoid or reduce the use of plastic wrap.
13. If you heat food in the microwave, use glass containers, since the heat tends to activate the release of chemicals present in the plastic. Keep in mind that even "BPA-free" plastics usually contain other endocrine disrupting chemicals as harmful as BPA.
14. Use glass feeding bottles for your baby.
15. Be careful handling purchase receipts. If you go to a store regularly, ask management for BPA-free receipts or have receipts sent by email.
16. Look for products that are made by ecologically sound companies that protect animals, are sustainable, certified organic and/or

are free of pesticides and GMOs. This applies to everything from food and personal care products to building materials, carpets, paints, baby items, furniture, mattresses, and more.

17. Choose toys made with natural materials and avoid plastic chemicals such as phthalates and BPA / BPS, especially on items that your child will likely suck on or bite.

18. Give your baby exclusively breast milk for at least the first year to avoid exposure to phthalates from baby formulas and nipples and pacifiers. There may also be pesticide contamination in baby formulas derived from GMO corn and soy.

19. Use natural cleaning products and if possible, make your own blends using natural ingredients.

20. Change personal care items, including shampoo, toothpaste, deodorants, and cosmetics, to organic alternatives.

21. Replace your vinyl shower curtain with a cloth product.

22. Replace feminine hygiene products (tampons and sanitary napkins) with safer alternatives; although most ingredients in feminine hygiene products are not listed on labels, many analyses suggest that they may contain dioxins and petrochemical additives, especially the more expensive ones.

23. Look for unscented products; phthalates are often used to help a product retain its fragrance longer; the artificial fragrance also contains hundreds of potentially toxic chemicals. Avoid fabric softeners, dryer wipes, inexpensive air fresheners, and cheap scented candles.

24. Check that household tap water is free of contaminants and filter water if necessary. It is also advisable to use an alternative to PVC pipes for water supply if that is applicable to your situation. Teach your children not to drink water from the garden hose, since many are made from plastic containing phthalates. Quality hoses are more expensive, but worth the investment.

25. It is important to ventilate the house as often as possible. Open the windows! It is an excellent way to live in a healthier home.
26. Seek and use safe, natural fragrances, candles, and room sprays.[1]

Ellen Sandbeck tells us, "No matter how polluted the outside air is, indoor air is often worse, due to the concentration of the gases emitted by modern amenities.[2]

For Further Reading Chapter 8

1. https://www.scientificamerican.com/article/toxic-perfumes-and-colognes/
2. https://books.google.com/books?id=AfvBaQaFtrcC&pg=PA286&lpg=PA286&dq=Sandbeck+tells+us:+%22No+matter+how+polluted+the+outside&source=bl&ots=zoOpDw5pyp&sig=y22cZJ-1eOjKcF5m2yBQehLcb3k&hl=en&sa=X&ved=0ahUKEwiwzYK6nNfRAhUJ8GMKHcL1DnEQ6AEIGjAA#v=onepage&q=Sandbeck%20tells%20us%3A%20%22No%20matter%20how%20polluted%20the%20outside&f=false

CHAPTER 9

Are There Natural Alternatives to Toxic Chemicals?

• • •

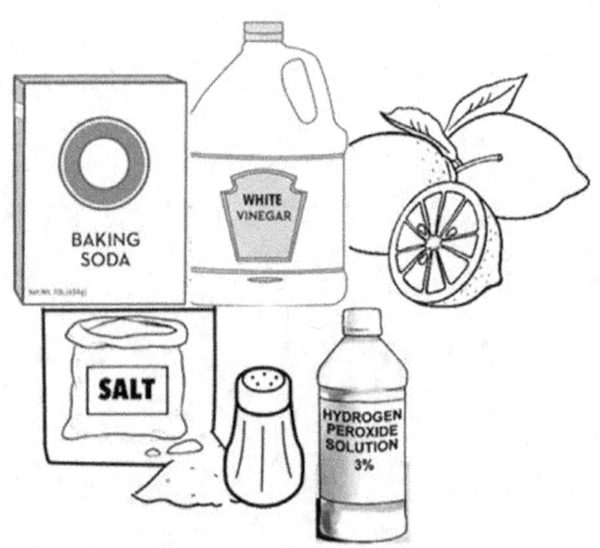

BAKING SODA

BAKING SODA IS ONE OF the most versatile ingredients in your kitchen. It is used to make bread and pastries and to remove bad odors from the refrigerator. It is present in beauty recipes, various medicinal uses and more. It is used for its abrasive power and deodorizing effects in domestic cleaning.

Uses for baking soda in cleaning the kitchen

Mix baking soda with water or place a small amount on a kitchen sponge (the sponge may contain kitchen soap as well) and you are ready to safely perform the following:

1. Remove the smell of food from your kitchen.
2. Remove coffee or tea stains.
3. Clean your microwave inside and outside.
4. Clean grease accumulations in your conventional oven.
5. Clean the inside and outside of your refrigerator.
6. Clean grease on your kitchen furniture and stove.
7. Clean your stove's surfaces including burners.
8. Disinfect and remove unpleasant odors from your chopping boards.
9. Clean your blender.
10. Clean knobs or controls without removing paint from the dials.
11. Remove stains from your dishwasher.
12. Clean food stuck on your pots and pans by boiling with baking soda and water.
13. Remove pesticides from your fruits and vegetables by washing with water and baking soda.
14. Clean glass doors of your cupboards and ovens.
15. Remove odors from your laundry by adding a little baking soda to your washing machine.
16. Add a small amount to of baking soda to toothpaste to facilitate whitening and plaque removal.
17. When taken internally, baking soda has been known to treat indigestion and heartburn.
18. Use baking soda as a powder for biopesticide control of fungal growth and termite reduction.

Read more here.[1]

Distilled White Vinegar

Distilled white vinegar is something that should be in every home. This product has many uses; it will save you time, money, and make your cleaning tasks easy and healthy. Although the smell of this product is not so pleasant, the results of using vinegar are impressive. It is fairly cheap, non-toxic, environmentally friendly, and can be used to do many things in the home. There has even been an announcement from Austria that the weed killer "Roundup" can be manufactured with vinegar as the active ingredient.[2]

Uses for vinegar in your home

Vinegar is a disinfectant and is bactericidal. Among other uses, it helps fade bad odors, remove stains, eliminate oxidation in metals, remove stains on carpets and cleans the coffee maker.

In addition, vinegar will:

1. Clean and disinfect your kitchen surfaces and bathrooms while making them shine.
2. Clean oxidized metal surfaces.
3. Rid surfaces of mineral deposits from hard water.
4. Clean your windows.
5. Bring a shine to your stainless steel, ceramic, plastic or chrome objects.
6. Clean and shine your mirrors.
7. Remove stains from your wooden furniture.
8. Clean and eliminate unpleasant odors in your bathrooms, kitchen, drains, and garbage disposal.
9. Eliminate the smell of cigarette smoke from your clothes by washing them with a small amount of vinegar or baking soda in the machine.
10. Eliminate wine stains on your clothing.

11. Prolong the life of your cut flowers.
12. Prevent ants from entering your house when sprayed at the base of your doors and Windows.
13. Eliminate the unpleasant smell in your house from pets.

Further reading is available here.[3]

LEMONS

Lemons are one of the most used condiments in cooking. Additionally, they are useful in cleaning your house. They are a true wild card that affords you a thousand cleaning solutions. Their fragrance is very pleasant; most people are fond of the aroma. Lemons can be used as the foundation material in ecological cleaning products or in air fresheners.

USES OF LEMONS FOR HOME CLEANING

Lemons also have a strong degreasing power that can be used in your kitchen and to eliminate difficult stains, like rust.

Lemons may also:

1. Eliminate unpleasant food odors in the kitchen.
2. Protect your iron when used with hard water.
3. Clean chopping boards in your kitchen.
4. Drive ants and cockroaches away due to its odor.
5. Freshen your linens when used in the wash.
6. Disinfect your kitchen utensils.
9. Eliminate scale from your bathroom faucets and kitchens.
10. Restore your metal kitchen utensils.
11. Eliminate grease from your cooking pans and utensils.

For further reading please go here.[4]

Salt

Thanks to its inherent properties, salt has been used from time immemorial to preserve or season foods. When used in normal doses, common salt is a versatile, abundant, economic, and generally, non-toxic substance, which makes it ideal for a number of your household tasks. Thanks to its chemical components, salt can be of great help solving many common cleanup issues in your home.

Uses of common salt to clean the home:

Salt's natural properties encourage its use as a natural food preservative. But it has many more uses. Salt is used to clean a multiplicity of surfaces. In your home, salt can be used alone or with other natural agents such as vinegar or lemon. Here are some suggested uses for salt.

1. Clean your kitchen table.
2. Clean up spills in your oven.
3. Clean your iron.
4. Remove coffee stains from your cups.
5. Remove rust spots on your clothing and textiles.
6. Remove burned grease stuck to your pots and pans.
7. Extinguish oil fires in your kitchen.
8. Keep your cut flowers fresh.
9. Control weeds even when in cracks.
10. Sprinkle salt to remove fleas from your house or pet.

To read more, I recommend this link[.5]

3% Hydrogen Peroxide

Hydrogen peroxide is considered to be the safest "natural" disinfectant and belongs in every home. It kills microorganisms by oxidation, which can be described as a controlled action process. When hydrogen peroxide reacts with organic material, it decomposes that material into oxygen and water. Most of us keep 3% hydrogen peroxide in our medicine cabinet just in case.

Cleaning your home and more with hydrogen peroxide

1. Used in your home, it is an excellent alternative to eliminate germs in place of toxic chemicals that are harmful to your health and the environment and leaves a fresh scent.
2. The antibacterial properties of hydrogen peroxide make it an excellent natural disinfectant to use both in your kitchen and in your bathroom.
3. Mixed with water, it can be used to clean glass and mirrors.
4. Disinfects your knives and various contaminated kitchen surfaces.
5. Disinfects your fruits and vegetables.
6. Disinfects your refrigerator and dishwasher.
7. Disinfects your kitchen sponges.
8. Cleans your pots and pans.
9. Whitens your clothes.
10. Removes mold.
11. Disinfects your toilet.
12. Disinfects toothbrushes.
13. Disinfects and cleans your floors.
14. Disinfects your children's toys.
15. Eliminates and avoids fungi in indoor plants.
16. Used topically it helps heal wounds.
17. Can be used for your oral health such as a mouthwash.
18. Prevents and combats fungus on your feet and nails.

You can read more about the uses of hydrogen peroxide here.[6]

For Further Reading Chapter 9

1. https://en.wikipedia.org/wiki/Sodium_bicarbonate
2. http://lactobacto.com/2017/05/23/roundup-made-with-vinegar-rather-than-glyphosate/
3. http://www.abowlfulloflemons.net/2013/02/10-ways-to-clean-with-vinegar.html
4. http://www.upsocl.com/verde/15-formas-de-utilizar-los-limones-que-probablemente-desconocias-y-deberias-probar/
5. http://modernsurvivalblog.com/remedies/30-uses-for-salt
6. http://www.naturallivingideas.com/hydrogen-peroxide-uses/

CHAPTER 10

Summing it All Up

• • •

During the course of preparing this book and its subsequent translation, steps have been initiated in Europe to regulate endocrine disruptors. As is usually the case, the pushback from industry has slowed progress and caused some divisive issues among some European Union member nations. The facts are, however, that humanity has been living with the presence of numerous kinds of toxic chemicals throughout most of the last century and changes to protect the health and the environment have always been slow. Consider the decade's long struggles to reduce/eliminate chemicals and substances such as artificial estrogens (Diethylstilbestrol, DES), cigarette smoke, PCBs, DDT, flame retardants, Bisphenol A, phthalates, the weed killer Atrazine, etc. Some are discussed here.[1]

Most recently (2017) we now are facing the influence of political decisions once again in the banning of an organophosphate insecticidal neurotoxin chlorpyrifos from use in the U.S. Despite the US EPA admitting risks exist to children and farm workers from exposures to this insecticidal neurotoxin in water and on crops, and numerous scientific studies showing chemical toxicity to children, this chemical is still in use after many years of legal actions to have it removed.[2]

This book was written with the good intentions of its author to educate the public and call attention to the issues posed by chemicals that all of us come in contact with daily. This daily contact combined with what is often delayed medical consequences of that exposure combine and make it extremely difficult to mount a credible concern about these toxic chemicals that are so common in our homes; but we are well past the breaking point. The technological soup of toxic chemical mixtures continues to grow, assaulting both our bodies and nature. We must do something to begin to reduce the incredible financial and personal health consequences of continuous exposures to such chemicals. During the last 50-75 years progress to eliminate the use of specific toxic chemicals has been slowed by court actions, ineffective and insufficient regulatory oversight, and influence from political perspectives without sufficiently relying on scientific evidence. To repeat, the United States philosophy of regulatory oversight does not rely on the precautionary principle (taking preventive action in the face of uncertainty) and this failure has led over the years to untold numbers of continuing medical cases and suffering of children, mothers, and the elderly.

The lack of knowledge on the part of citizens and consumers about the toxic chemicals in the products they use has also created a "hidden" emergency and furthers complacency. Some scientists consider the consequences of exposure to endocrine disruptors as a silent epidemic of worldwide proportions. These endocrine disruptors cause serious damages to the health of living beings and the environment. Recently, scientists have given a quantitate essence to the urgency and impacts of these exposures to endocrine disruptors by estimating annual medical and work lost impacts. These figures amount to hundreds of billions of dollars of costs annually in both Europe and the United States. The societal consequences of living with so many chemicals in our homes can only be resolved through massive public educational efforts and changes in lifestyle, greater safety in commercial everyday products from industry, and a stronger regulatory oversight and action taken by our elected officials and regulatory scientists in our government.

FOR FURTHER READING CHAPTER 10

1. https://www.ewg.org/release/ewg-lists-top-ten-toxic-chemicals-epa-should-review-now#.WgIahGhSxPY
2. https://earthjustice.org/features/what-you-need-to-know-about-chlorpyrifos

BIBLIOGRAPHY

• • •

In addition to the websites cited throughout the text, the following includes a few of the references used in the preparation of this book.

Books.

1. Harte, John. *Guide to Pollutants: The Toxic Book from A to Z.* S.A. Grijalbo, 1995.
2. Carson, Rachel. *Silent Spring.* Houghton Mifflin Co. New York, 1962.
3. Babich, M.A. *The Risk of Chronic Toxicity Associated with Exposure to Disononyl Phthalate (DINP) in Children's Products.* Report of U.S. Consumer Product Safety, Washington, D.C. 1990.
4. Colburn, T., Dumanoski, D., Myers, J.P. *Our Stolen Future. Do Synthetic Chemicals Threaten our Fertility, Intelligence and Survival?* The Penguin Group, New York. 1997.
5. Carey, F.A. *Organic Chemistry.* McGraw-Hill Interamerica of Spain. 2007.

Websites.

*Note: An English translation is often provided where the original article is in Spanish.

1. Theo Colborn. 2017. The Endocrine Disruption Exchange. Partners in Science. Retrieved from: https://endocrinedisruption. org/interactive-tools/endocrine-basics

2. Megana, F. 2014, March 24. *Experts Warn of New Chemicals that May Harm a Child's Brain Development.* Retrieved from http:// econcientiza.blogspot.com/2014/03/expertos-alertan-de-nuevos-quimicos-que.html

3. Women's Voices for the Earth. *Common Antimicrobial Chemicals Found in Household Sanitizers.* Retrieved from http://www. womensvoices.org/en-espanol/desinfectantes/

4. Emily Main. 2013, November 4. The 12-most toxic chemicals in your home. Retrieved from. https://www.prevention. com/health/healthy-living/top-12-endocrine-disrupting-chemicals-in-your-home

7. Márquez, Eva María Moreno and Azucena Núñez Álvarez. 2012. *Endocrine Disruptors, a Possible Toxic Risk in Products of Habitual Consumption.* Retrieved from http://hdl.handle.net/10272/6143

8. Megana, F.2014, February 19. *Expert Concerns About Chemicals Contained in Food Packaging.* Retrieved from http://econcientiza. blogspot.com/2014/02/preocupacion-de-expertos-por-sustancias. html

9. de Prada, Carlos. 2013. *Home without Toxics. How to Prevent Diseases by Eliminating Domestic Poisons.* Retrieved from www. hogarsintoxicos.org

10. Vidales, Raquel. 2013. *Are Air Fresheners More Toxic than Tobacco?* Retrieved from http://sociedad.elpais.com/sociedad/2013/09/26/ actualidad/1380212230_805033.htm

11. Schwart, Larry. 2016. *Toxic Traps: When These 7 Types of Plastics Are Dangerous. AlterNet.* Retrieved from http://www.alternet.org/

personal-health/toxic-traps-when-these-7-types-plastic-are-dangerous

12. *Hispantv. 2013 World Health Organization Warns of Hormonal Disorder Generated by Chemicals.* Retrieved from http://www.hispantv.com/noticias/salud/141802/oms-avisa-de-trastorno-hormonal-generado-por-productos-quimicos.

13. Yahoo Health. 2015 *Can Makeup And Cleaning Products Really Mess With Your Hormones?* Retrieved from https://www.yahoo.com/beauty/can-makeup-and-cleaning-products-really-mess-with-112897292102.html

14. Meeker, John, D. 2012. Exposure to Environmental Endocrine Disruptors and Child Development. Retrieved from https://www.ncbi.nlm.nih.gov/pmc/articles/PMC3572204/

15. Sigurdson, Tina. 2014. *Expert Panel Confirms that Fragrance Ingredient Can Cause Cancer.* Retrieved from http://www.ewg.org/enviroblog/2014/08/expert-panel-confirms-fragrance-ingredient-can-cause-cancer#.WZCq0a3MzdQ

16. Mozo, D. R. (2012) *Endocrine Disruptors: New Answers for New Challenges.* Retrieved from https://saludsindanio.org/articulos/americalatina/disruptores-endocrinos-nuevas-respuestas-para-nuevos-retos

17. Soto, Ana M. 2002.*Endocrine Disruptors: A Very Personal Story with Multiple Personalities.* Sanitary Gazette. Retrieved from http://scielo.isciii.es/scielo.php?script=sci_arttext&pid=S0213-91112002000300002

18. de Prada, Carlos. *Household Contamination Risks.* (2012) *The Chemical Epidemic.* Retrieved from https://www.casadellibro.com/libro-la-epidemia-quimica/9788496851580/2006319

19. Gonzales, A. (2014) *Working with Chemicals.* Retrieved from http://es.hesperian.org/hhg/Where_Women_Have_No_Doctor:El_trabajo_con_sustancias_qu%C3%ADmicas

WHAT READERS ARE SAYING ABOUT "LIVING WITH THE ENEMY."

• • •

JULIA SEIDLER'S BOOK, *LIVING WITH The Enemy*, takes the reader by the hand on a journey through the countless toxic chemicals that infiltrate our body. From beauty products to home décor to children's toys and with a focus on endocrine disrupting chemicals Seidler tells the hard truth about how we are causing great harm to our heath with the very products we use to clean and beautify our homes, our bodies, and our faces.

Read the book. Embrace the information. Make some easy changes. Improve your life.
. . . . . K.S.P., Author, Environmental Justice Writer, Communications coach

The author, Julia Seidler achieves her goal of alerting parents and all con-sumers about the hidden dangers of encountering toxic chemicals in every day products. Ms. Seidler reminds us all that there are direct interactions between our health and toxic chemicals in fragrances, furniture, cleaning products, garden products, food, electronics and more. Her point leads us to the conclusion that toxicology and healthy development must be the next frontier of medical and scientific research. Reading this book will invigorate you to take simple and effective steps to reduce toxic chemicals in your life.
. . . . L.A., Beyond Toxics

Even seasoned activists who work diligently to remove toxins from our environment, can learn a huge amount about the dangerous chemicals in our homes and offices with this heavily researched yet easily understandable book. This is a book for our times. It alerts us to the many toxic products found in toys, fragrances, pacifiers, furniture and more that may seem benign but are actually the cause of over $300 billion dollars a year of missed work and medical costs within the U.S. Julia Seidler ends the book with a useful list of twenty-six ways to reduce the dangers around us by using natural, inexpensive, non-toxic products.

. . . . .C. F., artist and activist

Can't wait to hold a class using Seidler's *Living with the Enemy*. It will change how we approach our household chores, gardening, and even our health and that of our children

. . . . D. W., Retired Librarian and Teacher

"Every consumer needs to read this book. Before you buy that next house, before you remodel that room, check out how to protect yourself from the many dangers that most are unaware of. Julia Seidler's book can guide you on how to provide a safer environment in your home. Buy it today and keep in on the reference shelf."

. . . . .M. M. Director of Oregonians for Safe Farms and Families

As a person more motivated when I know **why** I should take actions, I appreciate that this book documents the facts about chemicals in the environment and **then** provides some very practical precautionary steps to take. Thank you, Julia Seidler.

. . . . . . .L. C. Educator and leader, "Southern Oregon Pachamama Alliance"

Living With The Enemy is a wake-up call for consumers. Where we feel safest (at home), we are at risk. Julia Seidler's book will inspire you to take steps to protect yourself and your family from the dangerous substances found in everything from toothpaste to toys.

....................................V. B. Retired teacher, interpreter

This book by Julia Seidler provides us with a comprehensive education-a gift to us-the public-as the government is not keeping us safe from these chemicals and we must take personal action to protect our human health.

.... L. S. dedicated environmentalist

As a legislative aide, I learned about chemical exposures in our daily lives through the vigorous debate happening over a bill that would force companies to publicly expose the presence of 66 known toxins in any children's products and cosmetics. Not everyone will work in the capital, but anyone can read Julia Seidler's book to get the same warning and awareness that I did.

.................J. M, Former Legislative Aide in Oregon State Senate

INDEX

• • •

P

pacifier 10,11,83,102

paint xvi,8,9,27,30,38,42,70,71,765,
83,87

Paraben(s) 43,44,49

Paracelsus xvii,61

PCBs 20,23,25,30,39,63,71,74,76,93

penalty 37

perfluorinated compounds 35,36

persistent chemicals 34,41

pesticide xvi,5,7,9,13,19,20,23,25,27,
39-41,44-47,50,52,57,59,62,
70-72,74-76,80,82,83,87

petroleum based 1,8,76

PFOA 35,36,37

phenol 3

phthalates 4,10,20,23,31,32,63,74,75,76,
82,83,93

physical and anatomical factors 55

pillows 33

plastics xvi,1,9,10,11,18,19,23,30,31,32,
33,40,42,70,82,83,88,99

polyurethanes 8

pollinators 7,45

pollutants 8,19,21,27,42,68,71,72,97

pollution 2,28,29

precautionary principle 74,94

pregnant 24,30,67,73,74,76

preservative 9,38,43,90

PVC 9,10,11,30,32,83

puberty 18,24,64

R

Randolph ,Theron 3

Recycling 11,31

reduce the dangers of chemicals 81

regulated 20,22,34,40

reproduction 15,42

respiratory system 3,52

S

safety xv,11,26,30,36,37,48,59,60,
94,97

salt 90

scientific studies 43,44,47,74,93

semen 23,43

sexual function 15

shellfish 5,13

skin 3,6,18,29,38,43,44,51,53-57,68

sleep 15,32

supergerms 7

surfactants 42,54

synthetic pesticide 7,44,45

systemic poisoning 56

T

technosphere xv

Teflon 35,36,37,48,49

temperature 54

testosterone 17,63

textiles 32,33,36,40,90

thyroid hormone 16,17,25,32,36,74

toothpaste 6,32,39,43,83,87,103